Moralising Poverty

Do we judge the poor? Do we fear them? Do we have a moral obligation to help those in need? The moral and social grounds of solidarity and deservedness in relation to aid for poor people are rarely steady. This is particularly true under contemporary austerity reforms, where current debates question exactly who is most 'deserving' of protection in times of crisis. These arguments have accompanied a rise in the production of negative and punitive sentiments towards the poor.

This book breaks new ground in the discussion of the moral dimension of poverty and its implications for the treatment of the poor in mature welfare states, drawing upon the diverse political, social and symbolic constructions of deservedness and otherness. It takes a new look at the issue of poverty from the perspective of public policy, media and public opinion. It also examines, in a topical manner, the various ways in which certain factions contribute to the production of stereotyped representations of poverty and to the construction of boundaries between 'insiders' and 'outsiders' in our society. Case studies from the UK and Italy are used to examine these issues, and to understand the impact that a moralising of poverty has on the everyday experiences of the poor.

This is valuable reading for students and researchers interested in contemporary social work, social policy and welfare systems.

Serena Romano is a Research Fellow at the Department of Social Studies, University of Naples Federico II, Naples, Italy.

Routledge Advances in Health and Social Policy

Moralising Poverty

The 'Undeserving' Poor in the Public Gaze

Serena Romano

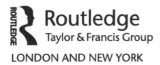

Routledge
Taylor & Francis Group

LONDON AND NEW YORK

First published 2018 by Routledge

2 Park Square, Milton Park, Abingdon, Oxfordshire OX14 4RN

52 Vanderbilt Avenue, New York, NY 10017

Routledge is an imprint of the Taylor & Francis Group, an informa business

First issued in paperback 2019

British Library Cataloguing in Publication Data
A catalogue record for this book is available from the British Library

Library of Congress Cataloging in Publication Data
A catalog record for this book has been requested

ISBN: 978-1-138-93978-3 (hbk)
ISBN: 978-0-367-34925-7 (pbk)

Typeset in Times New Roman
by Taylor & Francis Books

To B., and to our long walks along the Thames Path

Contents

Figures

Acknowledgements

This volume was produced during 2014 and 2016, and I owe my profound gratitude to many persons who helped me, at different institutions and in different places. It is a long list that includes first and foremost Professor Enrica Morlicchio, Professor Enrica Amaturo and all my colleagues at the Department of Social Studies in Naples for their constant support and confidence in my projects. A significant part of this book was written during a stay at Nuffield College, University of Oxford, through a Jemolo Fellowship, for which I would like to thank the Warden, Sir Andrew Dilnot, and my sponsor, Professor Erzsébet Bukodi. I am especially grateful to my colleague Virginie Tournay for very productive discussions at our breakfast table, but most of all for her kind support through a most difficult time. I am also indebted to Professor Margaret Greenfields at the Institute for Diversity Research, Inclusivity, Communities and Society (IDRICS) and Professor Tim Middleton for providing a stimulating environment and resources at Buckinghamshire New University. Special thanks also go to the editorial staff at Routledge for their great work and patience with my submission deadlines, and to several friends who provided help and logistic support during my field work in Naples and London.

I owe the greatest debt of gratitude to my fiancé Aldo for his continuous practical, intellectual, and psychological support, and for never allowing me to give up on this project. Finally, I want to thank my parents and grandparents for all the sacrifices they have made to help me with my work, and my sister Eleonora for taking very good care of our dog during my absence.

Man is only a moral being because he lives in society, since morality consists in solidarity with the group, and varies according to that solidarity. Cause all social life to vanish, and moral life would vanish at the same time, having no object to cling on.

Émile Durkheim, *The Division of Labour in Society*, 1893.

1   Introduction

The undeserving poor: those who are not excused

Human beings 'function as cognitive misers' (Massey, 2007: 9). We tend to think in 'categorical terms' and to construct general *schemas* through which we can easily classify, interpret and thus understand the world around us. The *deserving/undeserving poor dichotomy*, one of the main subjects of this book, is but one of the binary schematic categorisations that help us decode and assess reality. However, it contains two distinctive traits: it is predominantly constructed on *moral boundaries* (Steensland, 2010) and has profound implications for the *actual* treatment of the 'objects' of the classification – the poor.

It could be argued that the notion of undeserving poor is the result of our society's paradoxical attempt at aiding those in need while, at the same time, limiting solidarity only to those who conform to social expectations in terms of deservedness and merit. The very existence of a category of claimants who are deemed not 'deserving' of social support is, in fact, a fundamental mechanism of most systems of redistribution. It is regulated by the general basic assumption that certain categories of individual can be 'morally excused from work' (Handler, 1993: 859) on account of their assumed vulnerable status or condition, thus qualifying as *worthy poor*, while others, notably those who are considered *responsible* for their own poverty, do not 'deserve' collective support. Historically, and at a very general level, the aged, sick and infirm – together with children and widows – would fall within the former category, while all other *able-bodied* individuals would belong to the latter group.

These categories and their social significance have been subject to profound transformations throughout the centuries, but the idea of undeserving poor has never disappeared completely. This might seem to be preposterously inconsistent with the very ideals and objectives of the most important redistributing institution in capitalist society: the welfare state.

Social policy programmes, in theory, are meant to enhance social inclusion and not exacerbate social divisions, let alone exclude those in a condition of need. Limiting solidarity only to the deserving ones might seem unfair; but – and this is the main rationale for this book – what does 'fair' mean? How narrow is the category of those 'excused from work' and how is this defined? Are social and political categorisations centred on ideas of 'deservedness' and solidarity informed by *morality alone* or are there other factors such as economic, political and social convenience? How do these ideas change across space and time?

In order to answer these questions, a clear explanation of the concept of 'undeserving poor' is necessary. At least two definitions can be provided, depending on the perspective used. Firstly, the term 'undeserving poor' may refer to those persons who are excluded from social insurance schemes and who, as a result, find themselves relying on residual and stigmatising social-assistance programmes. According to Aaronson (1996: 214), this is the general rule in the US, where 'welfare is, in short, what happens to individuals whom we perceive as the undeserving poor'. This notion is strictly linked to the identification of welfare programmes with social assistance (or 'social welfare') schemes, predominantly used in the US. The second and most common interpretation of the undeserving poor as a concept is centred on the *complete exclusion* of certain categories of claimants from the system of public relief. Understood in these terms, the 'undeserving poor' notion contains both a *normative* and a *descriptive* element.

From a normative point of view, the undeserving poor category includes all those who *should not* be eligible for welfare benefits (regardless of whether they actually receive the payments or not) because their behaviour, condition or socio-economic characteristics are considered unworthy of public support. From a descriptive perspective, the term undeserving poor indicates those who are not part of the welfare system, precisely because of the aforementioned factors. Looking at the transformations of social policy and solidarity actions from the perspective of the undeserving poor is a powerful and fascinating sociological lens for our discussion. The contradiction regulating society's attitude towards the poor (which reads: only the worthy, deserving ones should be helped) is a fundamental mechanism not only of welfare systems but also of society in general. It can be argued, as Gans (1994) does, that if the undeserving poor continue to exist as a social phenomenon today, it is exactly because they perform a number of 'useful functions' in society, albeit to the exclusive advantage of the non-poor population.[1]

The first and most predictable function is an *economic* one. Welfare budgets are intrinsically limited and so is the capacity of states to protect their needy citizens, the result being that priority is given to those who pass the 'deservingness' test, be it explicitly formulated or implicitly assumed in the eligibility rules regulating social assistance programmes.

Secondly, the undeserving poor – meaning those who fail to demonstrate their efforts in fulfilling a given society's expectations – are a strong *societal* instrument of social cohesion for the non-poor population. Welfare policy, Handler and Hasenfeld remind us, is part of a 'moral system' that first defines 'who are the deviants' for the dominant groups, and then excludes and stigmatises them as the system's outcasts (1991: 12, 16). The exclusion of undeserving claimants from actions of solidarity and relief is thus, first and foremost, a 'societal reminder' of acceptable social values and modes of behaviour and an instrument of *norm reinforcement* for society as a whole. Moreover, the undeserving poor constitute convenient public 'cathartic objects' of scapegoating (Gans 1994: 272) in times of social, moral and economic crisis.

Thirdly, the presence of undeserving poor, and the rhetoric around them, may perform an action of *ideological* legitimisation of the political agenda. Negative representations and stereotyped classifications of the undeserving poor based on their alleged irresponsible and deviant behaviour can validate political narratives centred on the need to cut down on their 'dependence' on the system and provide *psychological relief* to the public for their exclusion from the welfare system.

Last, but no less important, deserving/undeserving dichotomies can also perform the function of *social control* by the welfare state, which *rewards* those who comply with the values and rules of the dominant group; *sanctions* (through exclusion from social policy programmes) those who fail to live in accordance with the said rules; and *influences* the behaviour of those who want to remain in the system.

Overview of the book

Having clarified one of the most important themes of our discussion, it is worth noting that this book does not concern itself merely with the undeserving poor; it also deals with the moral and social backgrounds of different societies' approaches to solidarity. As such, it intends to augment the existing literature on the moralising dimension of poor relief and solidarity, and discuss the relationships between poverty, social policy, media and public opinion. Three predominant questions underpin this study:

- Is *deservedness* as a dimension a universal, recurrent and constant component of poor relief actions?
- How do the cultural, economic and social characteristics of a given country impact on the construction of public solidarity and its underlying moral discourses in different contexts?
- Do stereotyped representations of the poor and negative attitudes towards the 'undeserving' welfare claimant emerge especially in times of (economic/political/social) crisis?

By providing both theoretical grounds and empirical evidence for the understanding of the moral dimension of solidarity and anti-poverty actions, with their multifaceted dynamics, this book breaks ground in support of the latter argument. In fact, the overriding argument of this work is that the moralisation, if not criminalisation, of the undeserving poor is a revolving element that occurs cyclically in societies – and especially so in times of 'moral panic'. Conceptualised by Stanley Cohen in his study on the sociology of deviance, moral panic is defined as the situation created when:

[a] condition, episode, person or group of persons emerges to become defined as a threat to societal values and interests; its nature is presented in a stylised and stereotypical fashion by the mass media. … Socially accredited experts pronounce their diagnoses and solutions. … Sometimes the object of the panic is quite novel and at other times it is something which has been in existence long enough, but suddenly appears in the limelight.

(Cohen, 1972 [2002]: 1)

The notion of 'moral panic' fits particularly well within the scope of this work as it perfectly summarises the main features of the public construction of the undeserving poor in times of social crisis. This notion will provide a fundamental analytical key to understanding the recurring exacerbation of hostility towards the undeserving poor in times of social and economic crisis. It will also help illustrate the extent to which, in some countries, the new wave of austerity measures triggered by the recent global economic crisis has restored the old stigmatising narrative centred on the deserving/undeserving dichotomy.

It is certainly true that, since the introduction of the very first poor-relief actions, governments have always been torn between whether to provide some relief to the poor, risking that welfare payment could 'undermine the will to work' (Flora, 1981: 343), or to deny it and face the threat of social disorder. However, in the past, the criminalisation of the undeserving poor was predominantly *physical*. Able-bodied individuals who failed to prove their willingness to work would either be banned from the community and imprisoned (as was the case for vagrants) or confined to the workhouse (especially after the seventeenth century). By contrast, as this book contends, contemporary forms of 'punishment' inflicted on the undeserving poor imply two main elements: their *exclusion* from public forms of relief – by means of stricter eligibility and conditionality rules required for access to social benefits; and the exacerbation of the *symbolic* moralisation, if not demonisation, of people reportedly undeserving of social protection, and their increasing public stigmatisation.

In this book, all these themes will all be examined from the multidimensional and cross-sectional perspective of morality. It is not by coincidence that the title of the book contains the term 'moral', which is inherently ambivalent, especially when associated with the word 'poverty'. Yet caveats should be made regarding the scope of our discussion: the reader will not find a systematic review of anti-poverty schemes, and experts in this particular domain may find the description oversimplified. Also, the volume itself is by no means a comprehensive account of poverty and its economic, social and psychological backgrounds. Rather, it looks at the relationships between morality, poverty and social inclusion/exclusion from three major standpoints:

- the 'moral dimension' of poor relief actions and solidarity;
- the public representation of the 'undeserving' poor and their alleged moral characteristics as depicted by the media and understood by public opinion; and

• the socio-cultural, moral and economic-based construction of boundaries between insiders and outsiders in our society.

Drawing the moral line: power, politics and culture

This book discusses the moral and social grounds of solidarity and deservedness in society. As such, it is concerned not solely with the representation and treatment of the 'undeserving' poor, but also with the overall relationships of solidarity and antagonism between the poor and the non-poor population. One of the most widespread misconceptions about anti-poverty policy is that it has always been a neglected domain of public policy, mostly uninteresting to the general public. Quite the contrary, historian Nicholas C. Edsall points out that before the advent of the modern welfare state, 'no body of legislation was of greater importance to the average [English]man than the laws for the maintenance and relief of the poor' (1971: 1): a 'considerable burden' in local taxes for the non-poor and the only possible form of relief distress for the destitute, he notes, poor legislation has always been at the centre of heated discussions.

Social reformer and influential member of the Fabian Society, Beatrice Potter Webb (together with her husband Sydney), was one of the first academics to provide a critical discussion of the 'continuously shifting and perpetually developing legal relationship between the rich and the poor, between the "Haves" and the "Have-nots"'. Her idea that the Poor Laws of the fourteenth and fifteenth centuries would deal not with the 'obligations of the rich to the poor' but with the 'behaviour of the poor to the rich' (Webb, 1928: 3) is somewhat illustrative of the optimistic view of the late Victorians that moral divisions between the poor and the non-poor were essentially a prerogative of pre-modern approaches to poor relief actions and of their faith in social progress. It is a fact that for a long time in the history of relief actions the poor, deserving and undeserving alike, have been subject to stigmatising and excluding 'othering' practices that weakened rather than empowered their social, economic and political rights, exacerbating their social division from the rest of society. The Victorian Poor Laws (1832) rule that denied middle-class men who received poor relief the right to vote is only too fitting an example of the multifaceted forms of social, political and economic mechanisms used to deter the public from using collective resources of support and, at the same time, of its divisive function in society. However, and despite the long tradition of poverty studies, the specific relationships between moral definitions/classifications, public policy design and the treatment of the poor in society are still unexplored, especially with regard to the processes through which deservedness is constructed, represented and legitimised.

Individualism vs solidarity?

In trying to fill the abovementioned gap in poverty studies, this book predominantly draws on original research material collected between 2014 and

2016. Although several sections of the book cover the moral backgrounds of poor relief and solidarity in general, the text is designed particularly to provide an in-depth analysis of Italy and the UK. Two emblematic cases of different approaches to poor relief and social inclusion actions – the Italian and British pathways and their current experiences – will guide us in our journey across the moral and social background of poverty relief and solidarity. There are a number of reasons for this particular comparison: for example, the lack of comparisons of this very kind in the existing literature, but most notably the alleged distance between these two countries in their experiences of poor relief and solidarity. Britain has been a pioneer in Europe in its adoption of formal legislation for poverty relief and, regardless of its approach, was indisputably the first country to assume the 'principle of public responsibility' for poverty, to quote Edith Abbott (1938: 260). In contrast, Italy has been one of the slowest of the industrialised countries to accept the role of so-called 'legal charity' and to institutionalise public solidarity for the poor. At the same time, Italy is generally looked at as the archetype of a social protection model centred on informal and 'spontaneous' channels of solidarity, first and foremost those provided through family and kin relationships, whereas the British model is often depicted as centred on an alleged culture of individualism and self-reliance. Investigating the roots of the apparent, almost mythical, opposition between the Catholic roots of a charitable and 'humanitarian' compassion and the 'disciplinary' state of poor repression is one underlying objective of this comparison. This book will illustrate that, in spite of their divergences in terms of outcomes, both countries present common characteristics, among which is the historical transition from the physical repression of poverty to its prevention. While the overall theme of the book is the moralisation of poverty, these two cases, with their different past and present approaches to poor-relief actions, provide an interesting key for analysing how different underlying cultures and moralities of solidarity may inform public policy actions and collective solidarity in different ways.

The moral and social bases of solidarity

An important aspect of this book is the resilience of moralising discourses on poverty and solidarity in the public sphere concerning political narratives, public opinion and the scientific world alike. The recurrent and cyclical re-emergence of knowledge frameworks centred on assumed distinctive traits on the part of the poor are perhaps the most indicative element of the never-ending story of their moralisation. Even in the second half of the twentieth century, for example, scientific accounts of poverty would frequently base their interpretations on assumed 'moral' and 'cultural' characteristics of the poor. One of the most popular sociological studies on the Italian social system, Edward Banfield's *The Moral Basis of a Backward Society*, advanced precisely this idea. Famously, Banfield attributed the diffusion of 'backwardness' and extreme poverty in the pseudonymous Montegrano – a small Italian village where he conducted his field work – to the villagers' 'inability to act together for their common good ... transcending the immediate, material interest of the nuclear family'. Such an inability, Banfield contended, was essentially derived from the population's 'cultural, psychological and moral conditions' and, in particular, from their inscribed 'ethos of amoral familism' (1958: 9–10). Similarly, but in a completely different context, Oscar Lewis's (1959) anthropological work on the relationship between poverty and an alleged 'subculture' of deviance among Mexican families is another example of the persistence, in contemporary times, of scientific paradigms centred on cultural and moral modes of behaviour of the poor and their assumed origin in the familial context.

It is true that, with critiques evidencing the limits of this stream of the literature in providing a comprehensive description of poverty and its main dynamics (Silverman, 1968; Muraskin, 1974), scientific paradigms centred on the role of 'morals' and 'culture' as determinants of poverty have almost disappeared over recent decades, making way for interpretations based on the effects played by other factors such as labour market exclusion, education, ethnicity, class, health, disability, gender, residential segregation, job insecurity and cumulative disadvantages, just to mention a few. However, by no means did the gradual (but never complete) disappearance of the 'moralisation of the poor' argument from the academic domain correspond to its elimination in *public life*. Political narratives justifying increasingly more selective approaches to social policy on the grounds of specific ideas of 'merit', 'deservedness' and 'equality' are a constant reminder of the underlying role of ethical frameworks in informing social policy interventions. Media representations of the undeserving poor, at the same time, do contain ethical judgements, which in turn affect and contribute to our ideas about social justice and deservedness.

One predominant question will drive our discussion over the following pages: can the diverse approaches and treatments of the poor (with their substantial outcomes in terms of inclusion/exclusion boundaries) be explained in terms of society's 'cultures' and 'moralities' of solidarity? To put it differently, we know for sure that at its 'prehistoric' stage (i.e. before the appearance of the modern welfare state), social policy legislations were profoundly imbued with moral and normative assumptions on the part of the non-poor population concerning assumed social characteristics of the poor, as well as with prescriptions on their expected behaviour. But is it still useful to look at the moral backgrounds of different social systems in order to understand their overall inclinations and attitudes to poverty and solidarity *today*? And, if this is the case, what is the role played not only by governments but also by society as a whole in the construction of a certain overall attitude towards the deservedness? This book postulates that these dimensions do indeed provide a fundamental analytical key for us to better understand different approaches to poverty at a societal level. In order to do so, we will reverse Banfield's and Lewis's idea that the moral and cultural backgrounds of the poor can explain poverty, and will try to provide an account of the 'moral and cultural bases' of different social systems and their role in the construction of distinctive approaches to poverty and solidarity.

An interdisciplinary study

Having clarified the main themes of the book, it should be evident at this point that such a discussion can only be accomplished through a multi-disciplinary lens. In this journey, not only sociology as a discipline, but also political science, media and urban studies will help shed light on the complicated social and moral construction of poor relief and solidarity actions in different societies. One of the principal assumptions of this work is that *societal beliefs, public policies* and *media representations* all contribute to the construction of specific social perceptions of welfare claimants, which, in turn, may affect the whole treatment of the poor population in a given society. An initial perspective considered in this work regards *social definitions*, societal beliefs and the role that social and moral categorisations play in the construction of different patterns of solidarity or exclusion, and in particular in the social production of the 'undeserving' welfare claimant as a category. Understanding the 'moral backgrounds' of a given society's view(s) on themes such as poverty, deservedness, solidarity and social justice is not only a matter for philosophical speculation.

At least since the appearance of the 'Thomas Theorem'- according to which 'If men define situations as real, they are real in their consequences' – sociology has revealed the power of social categorisations in constructing and reinforcing reality (Thomas and Thomas, 1928: 572). Stigma, which for sociologist Erving Goffman is a discrediting attribute of *differentness* around physical, moral or tribal characteristics that the 'normals' assign to 'others', is always the product of a social categorisation process (Goffman, 1963: 2–5, emphasis added). This process begins with the construction of a 'virtual social identity', that is, a characterisation of the (stigmatised) individual made by means of imputations; but it can end up with very real consequences in terms of the 'moral career' and experiences available to those living with the stigma (ibid.: 32–33). As such, not only do moral definitions, categories and classifications constitute one of the fundaments of social interactions, but they are also profoundly embedded in different realms of the public sphere.

Above all, as this book will illustrate, these categorisations are a predominant element of social policy, which intrinsically 'both responds to and produces moral categories in society' (Steensland, 2010: 455). This applies particularly within public actions directed towards the poor. Georg Simmel, perhaps the first author to recognise that poverty is socially constructed, demonstrated that this phenomenon 'cannot be defined in itself as a quantitative state, but only in terms of the social reaction' that it provokes. By arguing that one cannot be said to be 'socially poor until he has been assisted' (Simmel and Jacobson, 1965: 138), Simmel encapsulated a fundamental aspect of contemporary poverty and social policy issues: the *mutual obligations* existing between the poor (to prove their condition of need) and their community (to help those in need) are necessarily imbued with moral judgements. In order to be 'socially recognised', and therefore assisted as such, the poor are obliged to give up their privacy and make their private life 'open to public inspection' and subject to strict scrutiny (Coser, 1965: 145) so that their *deservedness* of assistance may by verified. This process, which applies overall to informal channels of solidarity and public policies alike, is epitomised by the construction of deservingness (Schneider and Ingram, 2005; Altreiter and Leibetseder, 2015) in contemporary welfare states, with their mechanisms and rules regulating eligibility and access to income support schemes, which are primarily those based on the implicit distinction between deserving and non-deserving claimants.

Finally, it is clear that the media plays a major role in the construction of poverty and its principal representations. A major assumption in most media and communication studies is that the information they provide is never neutral and objective, but always presented to the public with specific connotations and meanings, the purpose being the transformation of the 'consciousness of the public' (Gamson et al., 1992; Terranova, 2004; Fuchs, 2011). Given their salient role in the construction of social realities, not only do the media contribute to the formation of public opinion and produce specific social and cultural portrayals of welfare claimants and the poor; they also act as filters and vehicles of transmission of the political narratives used by governments to legitimise their moral and political orientations around poverty to mould public opinion. It goes without saying that the pivotal role that the media play in the propagation of ideologies, norms and values produced by dominant groups is of fundamental significance to our discussion (Hall, 1980). By devoting attention to specific aspects of poverty, or to distinctive categories or modes of behaviour of welfare claimants, the media can significantly influence public attitudes and sentiments on these matters. They may also, as a number of studies have shown, perpetrate erroneous assumptions concerning welfare recipients and stereotypical images of the poor (Gilens, 1996; Clawson and Trice, 2000). These three elements (social categorisations, public policies and media representations) all play their part in the construction of a society's approach to poverty and solidarity. Together they form a complicated nexus that ultimately produces the dominant representations and treatment of poverty, together with the stigma that is frequently attached to the condition of 'undeserving poor'.

Structure of the book

As mentioned in the previous section, in this work the moral dimension of poverty is addressed from three primary standpoints:

- the 'moral dimension' of public and social policy;
- the public representation of the 'undeserving' poor and their alleged moral characteristics as depicted by the media and public opinion; and
- the cultural, political and power-based construction of boundaries between insiders and outsiders in our society.

In accordance with the three-fold aim of the study, the book is divided into three parts, each of which is dedicated to one of the above-mentioned areas of analysis. Part I provides a conceptual and historical framework for the understanding of the leitmotif of the study – the moral treatment of the poor in our society – with a special, albeit not exclusive, emphasis on Italy and the UK. Chapter 2 retraces the origins of the concept of deservedness in western societies and its evolution over time from the perspective of three recurring themes in public actions directed towards the poor: idleness, deviance and discipline. Chapter 3 looks at the social and moral background of welfare programmes and solidarity in Italy and Great Britain. Chapter 4 discusses the emergence of a moralising discourse in the welfare state in conjunction with the Great Recession.

A second major perspective from which the moral dimension of poverty is addressed in Part II takes into consideration the public and symbolic representation of poverty in a broad sense. Chapter 5 describes the increasing attention devoted by the general public to the undeserving poor and the emergence of a number of 'mythological' figures such as the 'welfare queen' in the US and the welfare 'scrounger' in Britain. Furthermore, it deals with the 'spectacularisation' of poverty and the role played by the media in the reproduction of stereotypes regarding the poor. Drawing upon data from the Eurobarometer and original material from focus group interviews, Chapter 6 discusses the case for a new wave of 'scroungerphobia' in Britain.

Part III discusses how the boundaries between *insiders* and *outsiders* are constructed in society, with special regard to solidarity. Chapter 7 explores the world of solidarity and spatial inclusion of immigrants in host societies, and raises the question of whether different geographies of solidarity exist in Italy and the UK. Drawing upon empirical material collected via semi-structured interviews with low-income migrant workers in Naples and London, this chapter examines the social construction of neighbourhood integration and community solidarity networks of immigrants. Chapter 8 further discusses the political and power-based construction of insider/outsider boundaries in Italian and British societies. It illustrates that the narrative based on the dichotomy between 'in-groups' and 'out-groups' in the welfare state is epitomised nowadays by scapegoating practices directed not only at 'undeserving' welfare claimants but also at immigrants and refugees. The chapter discusses how these attacks on the 'stranger' can be best understood as a reaction to emergency situations, of which the latest refugee crisis and the Brexit result are but two examples.

Note

1   Gans lists 13 'useful functions', which he divides into four macro categories: social, economic, moral and political.

Part I

The moral background of poor relief and solidarity in public policy

2 The origins of deservedness: idleness, deviance and discipline

Framing the issue: the 'moral factor'

In one of the most important studies on poverty and the welfare state, Piven and Cloward famously stated that the whole history of anti-poverty policy is essentially a record of 'periodically expanding and contracting' relief actions through which the system performs two main functions: maintaining civil order and enforcing work (1971: xvii). While there is wide agreement in the scientific community on the *disciplining* component of poor relief actions, comparative and even national accounts of social policy have generally failed to retrace how the above-mentioned functions of poor relief change from one context to another, and to centre their investigations on the moral and social backgrounds of public policies aimed at the poor. Despite increased interest in the ethical fundaments of welfare regimes and social policy programmes (Applebaum, 2001; Chunn and Gavigan, 2004; Schneider and Ingram, 2005; Saunders, 2013; Altreiter and Leibetseder, 2015) and in the moral dimension of poverty alike (Galston et al., 2010; Spicker, 2007; Weiner et al., 2011), morality in the welfare state remains largely unexplored as a domain, with only a few – and regrettably outdated – exceptions (Katz, 1990 [2013]; Dean, 1991; Handler and Hasenfeld, 1991; Himmelfarb, 1991; Frey and Morris, 1993).

This chapter is precisely dedicated to discussing the moral foundations of poor-relief actions before the advent of the modern welfare state. Following Leiby (1985: 323), we can define these foundations as the 'general rationale offered for any and every sort of social welfare activity' which are 'part of the religious and political beliefs and attitudes of our culture'. In addressing this theme, two major theoretical frameworks stand as fundamental milestones guiding our discussion. First and foremost is the notion of *moral economy* in its broad conceptualisation. Historian E. P. Thompson coined this expression in support of his argument that the food riots in eighteenth-century England were not triggered merely by rising prices and hunger. Rather than 'rebellions of the belly', he pointed out, these tumultuous events occurred because the *social consensus* over the moral obligations of the ruling class towards the poor was broken. In fact, it was the whole legitimacy of the underlying 'old moral economy of provision' that was called into question by the population, together with the overall acceptance that 'any man should profit from the necessities of others ... in times of dearth' (Thompson 1971: 77, 132).

Thompson's remained for a long time one of the few comprehensive studies to highlight the ambivalent relationship between public opinion, consensus, morality and solidarity.[1] It was only in the 2000s that another major study on this topic emerged with Steffen Mau's work on the moral economy of welfare state institutions. Deriving precisely from Thompson's insights on the moral implications of economic behaviours and their legitimisation processes, Mau's study has paved the way for a new understanding of the normative dimensions of public policy actions. More importantly to the discussion made in this volume, it evidenced that poor-relief actions, and in general public support for those in need, always contain a 'moral dimension'. As reciprocal exchanges that must be legitimised and made 'plausible' to the eye of the public, welfare and social transactions are necessarily grounded upon a 'constituted and subjectively validated set of shared moral assumptions' (Mau, 2003: 31).

The main theme of this chapter is the 'moral factor' argument regulating poor relief and solidarity actions before the advent of the modern welfare state. Fabian reformers Sydney and Beatrice Webb (1910, Webb and Webb, 1911) were probably the first academics to use this term in a critical manner when they admitted the importance of the moral 'defect' of the individual contributing to his/her destitution but, at the same time, warned against the use of instruments of deterrence to discipline the poor on the grounds that moral failure may not always be 'in those who are destitute', but rather in the actions of other individuals or of the community itself. The very fact that this position was held by two of the most progressive reformers of their time is only too indicative of the ambivalent yet recurrent role of morality as a universal component in public policy.

Irrespective of being latent or open, not only is the distinction between deserving and undeserving categories of welfare claimants commonly found in every society (Katz, 1990; Saraceno, 2002; Lister and Bennett, 2010) but it also constitutes the very foundation of each welfare state and its 'perpetual dilemma': that of providing citizens with generous welfare programmes (and low work incentives) as opposed to the minimal social protection (and high levels of inequality) option (Saunders, 2013). This dilemma is generally resolved precisely by what could be termed the *selective generosity* alternative: that is, by regulating that *only* certain categories of needy claimants (namely those assessed as deserving of social protection) may be eligible to receive social protection. However, if deservedness can be said to be the solution to the perpetual dilemma of modern welfare states, the very idea that poor relief and social support should be 'deserved' has been at the centre of philosophical and political discussions for centuries now. But where *exactly* can we trace its origins? In the following sections, we will search for the roots of a deservedness idea in public policy from the perspective of three, apparently unconnected, elements: *idleness, deviance* and *discipline*.

The moralisation of idleness in the western world

The nexus between morality, poverty and public policy is nothing new. It is generally assumed that the emergence of the whole 'deservedness' discourse in poor-relief actions coincides with the establishment of the welfare state, or at least with its 'prehistoric' phases (Flora and Heidenheimer, 1976: 22), back in the days of the English Poor Laws, with the workhouse system fulfilling the aims of separating the deserving and undeserving poor into two distinctive social, economic and moral categories. In reality though, the emergence of a moralising element in public policy can be traced back even further, surprisingly enough to the birth of democracy in ancient Greece and its ambivalent approach to the idea of 'idleness'.

Equality and the moral condemnation of idle individuals were two apparently contradictory but characteristic cornerstones of Athenian society at the time of Pericles (460–429 BC). Among the several reforms that made Athenian democracy and citizenship flourish under his leadership, Pericles' original solution to the problem of destitution and unemployment is perhaps the more indicative of these two cornerstones.[2] Driven by the concern that 'common labourers should neither have no share at all in the public receipts, nor yet get fees for *laziness* and *idleness*',[3] Pericles suggested employing them in great construction projects, which made him the most eminent precursor of Keynesianism (Lewis, 1992: 139), and possibly the first advocate of workfare schemes in the western world. At the same time, Pericles sent thousands of poorer Athenian citizens (the *thetes*) to settle in overseas colonies, named *cleruchies* (Glotz, 1926). The two-fold role of cleruchies as both military outposts and a means of social engineering is strikingly illustrated by Plutarch, who described Pericles' decision as mainly driven by the aim of 'lightening the city of its mob of lazy and idle busybodies, rectifying the embarrassments of the poorer people'.[4]

Ancient Rome seemingly shared with Athens a similar ambivalent approach towards poor-relief actions and deservedness. Almsgiving was generally approved and actually considered a duty, and the highest expression of human *virtus*. The practice of providing free (or subsidised) wheat to the poor (i.e. the vast majority of the population at that time), referred to as *grain dole*, survived across centuries – and even became hereditary (Haskell, 1939; Garnsey, 1988; Aldrete, 1994). However, at the same time as feeding the poor, these institutions nourished a certain stereotyped and negative representation of the 'wheat mob' (*plebs frumentaria*) as an idle and lazy collective who would rely on the state for their own immoral life (Morley, 2006). Needless to say, this view, which was very popular among the Republic's intelligentsia, was imbued with moral judgements and ethical prescriptions, as Cicero's caveat reminds us: charity must always be 'deserved', that is, it must be done 'according to the recipient's merit', behaviour and 'moral character'.[5] In the latter days of the Empire, the very decadence of the Republic came to be attributed by contemporaries exactly to the idle lifestyle of the mob, concerned only with its appetite for 'bread and circuses', as popularised by the satirist Juvenal.

Another, fundamental milestone in the development of an ambivalent moralising approach to poverty and idleness in the western world lies within the Christian tradition, and more precisely encapsulated in Saint Paul's admonition in the Bible, which reads:

> We command you, brothers and sisters, to keep away from every believer who is idle and disruptive [...] for we gave you this rule: the one who is unwilling to work shall not eat.[6]

This quotation, which strikes us as something apparently in utmost contrast with the Christian ethics of charity, piety and solidarity and the moral obligation to help the poor,[7] has found a number of different interpretations and explanations in the literature (for a discussion see Van Til, 2010). The ambivalent relationship existing between poor-relief actions and moral prescriptions regulating the behaviour of the needy – first and foremost the elimination of indolence and laziness among them – draws a line of continuity between Pericles' and Cicero's visions and Saint Paul's words, which is far from accidental. In this regard, Helen Rhee's recent study (2012) is enlightening in its illustration of how early Christians appropriated the Greco-Roman 'moral teaching' and practices regarding poverty and the poor, and transformed them in accordance with their new ethical frameworks, most notably those concerning the spiritual use of almsgiving as a *redemptive* action.

Others, most famously Max Weber, understood Saint Paul's words as the utmost expression of the *Protestant ethic*, which incorporated that principle and made labour per se 'the end of life', thus considering 'unwillingness to work [as] symptomatic of the lack of grace' (Weber, 1930 [2005]: 105). Perhaps even more importantly to our discussion, Weber notoriously evidenced that, among the several transformations that it brought about, the Protestant Reformation also marked a profound watershed in the Christian cultural approach towards the ethics of work. Medieval interpretations of Saint Paul's above-mentioned precept would emphasise the role of labour as a natural necessity for humanity in general, whereas puritan theologians came to understand it as a *moral warning* against idleness. As an ascetic technique against all temptations, work was exalted by Lutherans and, in fact, prescribed as a duty for *all* individuals without exception. Weber's intuition and his line of argumentation have been further expanded by contemporary scholars' accounts of the allegedly different visions of work and poverty in the Catholic and Protestant worlds. For some time, the predominant argument in this regard has been that, besides producing two distinct approaches to the ethics of work, the Protestant schism from the Roman Catholic Church also played a significant role in the consolidation of two diverse social and moral approaches towards poverty and poor-relief actions, with Protestant countries (such as Britain, the Netherlands and the United States) becoming more inclined than Catholic nations (including Italy, France and Spain) to create a social and moral separation of the poor into two different categories – namely the 'worthy' and 'unworthy' poor.

Historiographical works of recent decades, however, have examined this view and called into question the assumed sharp opposition between the 'sentimental' approach to solidarity and charity assigned to the Catholic Church (Pullan, 2005: 446) and the Protestant world of poor relief actions (Dean, 1991). In fact these studies showed the two approaches were very similar in their ambivalent treatment of the poor, with almsgiving and the punishment of the poor being two sides of the same coin in both cultures (McIntosh, 2012). More pertinent to the present discussion, this literature suggested that public policy in both the Catholic and the Protestant worlds has been found articulated around the division of 'deserving' and 'undeserving' poor into two separated social and legal categories (Pullan, 1976).

Even within this stream of the scholarship, however, it is conceded that it would be erroneous to understand the Catholic approach to the care of the poor as *casual* and to forget the 'transcendental aims of most charitable actions' Pullan, 1976: 33). Rather, the religious element can be understood as one aspect of the complex socio-economic, political and legislative nexus of solidarity and poor-relief actions in different contexts. We could accept in this regard Kahl's view (2005) that looking at the roots of diverse 'social doctrines' (with their diverse religious fundaments) can help the investigation and understanding of contemporary cross-national variations in poverty policy.

Equally important to our investigation is the role played by the moral frameworks of legislators and governors. If, as Spicker (2013b: 189) evidences, governments are 'moral actors' because their 'decisions and actions are informed by moral considerations' and they 'carry moral responsibility for the decisions they make', then it seems appropriate to assume that the approaches of early modern European legislators to poverty and poor relief actions would be informed and affected by ethical considerations (including religious beliefs), as is the case with their contemporary counterparts today (Grell et al., 1999). For example, although negative sentiments against idleness have always existed, as discussed above, it is perhaps no coincidence that the exaltation of the imperative to work and the exacerbation of a moral hostility against laziness in England found its culmination precisely after the Reformation under the reign of Elizabeth I, who is generally reported as the first to have formalised the distinction between 'deserving' and 'undeserving poor'. As a matter of fact, such a separation, as the next section illustrates, has characterised most public policy approaches to idleness, almsgiving and vagrancy in early modern Europe. It is a truism, however, that, even more than any other Protestant movement in Europe, the Elizabethan Anglican Church embraced entirely the new ethic of labour and expanded it significantly, predominantly as a consequence of the gradual elimination of ecclesiastic poor relief actions implemented at the local level and their substitution with private charity and public policy. There is no doubt that the transposition of social hostility against idleness into law would have a profound influence in the development of the overall political and social approach to poor relief and solidarity in the Anglo-Saxon world – which, arguably, differs significantly from the route taken by Catholic countries.

'V' is for vagabond

The previous section briefly introduced the theme of idleness as an assumed moral condition 'attached' to poverty, and as a recurrent theme in the history of public policies aimed at the poor. It has illustrated the extent to which moral judgements regarding distinctive behaviours and attitudes of the poor are almost as old as humanity. Most notably, suspicion of and antipathy towards idleness and inactivity have always existed as fundamental counterparts to most societies' approaches to solidarity, charity and poor relief actions. In order to further our discussion on the moral backgrounds of poor relief actions in public policy and the construction of the undeserving poor as a social category we must now introduce a second element of analysis: deviance.

If moral decadence can be said to have been commonly understood as the predominant *cause* of idleness and inactivity among the poor for centuries, the links between poverty and crime have always been much more ambiguous and thus highly debated even in the scientific community, with a part of the scholarship postulating that a direct cause–effect relationship exists between poverty and crime and others maintaining that the inverse is true. The literature on the association of crime and poverty is thus extremely rich, and has produced several different accounts of the supposed interconnections between disadvantaged environments, poverty, culture and criminal behaviours, all of which cannot be taken into full account here. The 'culture of poverty' theory formulated by anthropologist Oscar Lewis in the 1960s is frequently mentioned as the first conceptualisation of the idea that a '(sub)culture' of social deviance exists in poor neighbourhoods which is absorbed by children, perpetrated in their behaviours and transmitted from generation to generation (Lewis, 1959). In fact, this idea and the predominant questions regarding the connection between poverty and social deviance that Lewis and other scholars pose are only the contemporary version of a historical preoccupation with the association of deviance, moral (mis)conduct and poverty, which finds its most visible roots in medieval times.

The long history of suspicion towards inactive persons as dangerous and deviant elements is exemplified by the overall criminal treatment of beggars and vagrants – the personification of idleness – and its transformation from the Middle Ages to modern times. Although a general rule applied across premodern Europe – that the beggar would be tolerated and the vagrant despised (Fontaine, 2014: 13) – a certain distinction between different categories of alms-seekers can be detected as early as the fourteenth century, far before the introduction of the English Poor Laws, when mendicants and vagabonds became the very first 'recipients' of the 'oldest continuous legal system of welfare relief in Europe' (Charlesworth, 2012: 53). One should be careful not to think of early poor laws in terms of proper anti-poverty programmes aimed at reducing marginalization and deprivation among the poor. In fact, at least until the early nineteenth century the history of poor legislation is essentially one of criminal laws aimed at relieving poverty in a 'framework of repression', as famously contended by Beatrice Webb (1928: 5), by means of harsh measures designed to punish the able-bodied wandering poor and mendicants as *offenders*.

Commonly reported as a direct social reaction to the Black Death of the previous year and the consequent labour shortages, the English Statutes of Labourers of 1349–1351 prohibited almsgiving to beggars who refused to work (Putnam, 1908; Chambliss, 1964; Geremek, 1987; Dean, 1991; Hatcher, 1994) on the grounds that charity would have acted as a disincentive to labour, increasing people's tendency 'to idleness and vice, and sometime to theft and other *abominations*'.[8] The moral and criminal *distinction* drawn between idle vagrants and the rest of the worthy population of 'impotent' poor – a predecessor of contemporary *selectivity* mechanisms in social policy – was predominantly based on an overall evaluation of their physical conditions, with only infirm destitute individuals being classified and treated as 'true subjects' or 'true beggars'. The wide range of punitive actions against 'sturdy' (i.e. fit to work) mendicants and vagabonds attest to the existence of a certain hostility against these groups in most European countries. These measures would include imprisonment (England, 1351), pillory and branding (France, 1351), perennial exile (Spain, 1540) flogging (Italy, 1596), enslavement, galley servitude and even the death penalty for inveterate offenders (England, 1572) (Martz, 1983; Rawlings, 2002; Weber and Bowling, 2008; Grell et al, 1999; Wardhaugh, 2000).

However, by the end of the sixteenth century the expansion of the beggar population in European cities – variously interpreted as a 'by-product of economic progress' (Aydelotte, 1913: 5), the result of the expropriation of agricultural people from the soil (Marx, 1887 [1976]) or as derived by the lack of local employment opportunities (Pound, 1971) – made the phenomenon of wandering 'masterless men' (Beier, 1985) extremely visible to the public eye, and further exacerbated the punitive approach to vagrancy. Marx himself described this process and the 'bloody' legislation against vagabondage in terms of a paradoxical development that came to 'chastise the fathers of the working class' for their *enforced mass* transformation into beggars (1887: 896).

Reportedly, this is especially evident in the case of post-Reformation England, where the criminalisation of idleness assumed the traits of a true 'penal semiotics' (Foucault, 1977; Carroll, 1996: 39). The practice of labelling officially licensed beggars with special badges that could positively distinguish them from 'counterfeiters' and fraudulent beggars was soon replaced by the *negative* identification of unworthy mendicants, who became criminalised and *literally* stigmatised. An English statute of 1547 ordered that idle able-bodied vagrants would be labelled as 'vagabonds' and branded with a hot iron with a 'V' on their chest (or with the letter 'R' for rogue) so as to make the mark on the idler 'a perpetual mark during his life' (Burn, 1764: 45). It is precisely in this practice that we can find the very essence of stigma in its original notion: 'a bodily sign designed to expose something unusual and bad about the *moral status* of the signifier' (Goffman, 1963: 1, emphasis added).

The exacerbation of anti-vagrancy legislation in this period is paralleled by the transformation of social and even visual representations of poverty. The description of vagrants as criminals and fraudsters became a recurrent exotic motif in the literature of early modern Europe (Hug, 2009; Woodbridge, 2001). Jütte (1994: 14) interestingly demonstrated that this shift is most visible when we compare images of the poor in the fifteenth and sixteenth centuries – with the former predominantly characterising paupers with physical deformities (most often they would be depicted as cripples) and the latter portraying them in a begging gesture – so as to underline that the main feature of the poor was not their physical status but rather their behaviour, and 'moral condition'.

As mentioned above however, even Catholic countries (including Italy) operated a certain distinction between the licensed worthy poor (generally the blind and crippled) and unworthy beggars (most notably 'alien' beggars), who would be subject to expulsion at the sign of any economic crisis. This occurred as early as the beginning of fourteenth century (Jones, 1997); but, as elsewhere in Europe, it was at the end of the fifteenth century, and in conjunction with the food and epidemic crises, that Italian legislators started to introduce a new approach to vagrants and beggars – which was to help those deemed deserving of assistance and punish the 'immoral' and recalcitrant undeserving poor (Black, 2001: 204).

In fact, the symbolic and corporal criminalisation of idleness was not only a matter of morals; it was also, and predominantly, a matter of social order. Above all, it was a necessary reaction to a 'public threat', with anti-vagabondage ordinances designed to contain and mobilise the increasing population of masterless wandering poor, especially those considered dangerous charlatans (Piven and Cloward, 1971).

Regardless of their social behaviour, supposed danger to society and moral conduct, under the anti-vagrancy laws framework recidivist vagabonds would become *de facto* proper felons, thus realising a self-fulfilling prophecy (Merton, 1948). This transformation can be understood as part of what Foucault (1977: 77) has described as the 'shift from a criminality of blood to a criminality of fraud'.

However, it is a truism that the symbolic and penal separation of worthy beggars from the 'fraudulent poor', which occurred even before the introduction of the Elizabethan Poor Laws, produced an 'opprobrium' against sturdy vagrants (Beier, 1974: 6) that must also have contained a moralising approach not only aimed at vagabondage and idleness but also at poverty as a phenomenon (Herrup, 1985; Tronrud, 1985; McMullan, 1987).[9]

To be sure, while officially aiming at disciplining the moral character of unworthy beggars and containing the deviant dangerous behaviour of potential fraudsters, the criminalisation of vagrancy also had an economic purpose – that of incentivising (if not forcing) labourers to accept low wages in a labour-shortage context (Chambliss, 2004). All in all, it can be argued that such an approach paved the way for a social definition of idleness as a *social and economic crime* and, at the same time, for the moralisation and disciplining treatment of 'unworthy', fit-to-work, adult poor for their decadence and assumed propensity to act as social deviants or even criminals.

Hotels, hospitals and prisons: the spatial dimension of discipline

A third element in our journey across the historical origins and developments of deservedness as a notion concerns the *disciplining* component of public policy: assistance and charity actions aimed at the poor, and in particular the spatial dimension of this element. Strictly connected to both the deservedness and deviance elements referred to above, the disciplining intent of poor relief actions is especially observable in the transformations introduced during the sixteenth and eighteenth centuries around Europe.

It is true, as illustrated in the previous section, that Christian and Protestant countries alike adopted a similar, generally unfriendly attitude towards 'unworthy' poor, vagrancy and idleness during the Middle Ages and early modern times. However, by the mid sixteenth century a new *social crisis*, predominantly produced by the widespread fall in real wages and the ongoing cycles of epidemics and food crises, made poverty and vagrancy 'the challenge of time' in most European countries (Geremek, 1994: 120). New solutions emerged, most notably the use of spatial *confinement* and *isolation* of the poor as an option to containing and educating them while reducing their visibility and setting them to work. Arguably, it is precisely in the formulation of these new strategies and in their underlying different intentions that perhaps one can find the origins of two distinctive 'cultures' of solidarity and support for the poor in both Catholic and Protestant countries. The different social and even *moral architecture* (Scull, 1980; Driver, 1993) in different contexts of places of physical discipline for the poor has proven, in fact, to be revealing of their relationships with the 'social aspirations, both religious and secular of those who erected them' (Pullan, 1995: 9).[10]

It is specifically in the comparison of the English and Italian cases, with their different approaches to the correction of the poor and to internment as a way to tackle poverty, that we can find further insights for our discussion of the social and moral backgrounds of solidarity and poor relief actions. By introducing local payment rates for the relief of the poor, the Elizabethan Acts promulgated during 1597 and 1601 (popularised as the 'Old Poor Laws') reportedly marked the introduction of a statutory 'social action' towards the relief of destitution in England (Himmelfarb, 1984: 188). The Acts codified the *duty* of all local parishes in England and Wales to help the 'Lame, Impotent, Old, Blind, and such other among them being Poor, and not able to work' who lived in the *same* parish,[11] although a right to receive such an assistance on the part of the poor was not formulated. Quite the contrary in fact: driven by the paternalistic assumption that poverty could be best addressed by 'correcting' the needy, the new law regulated that the duty of parishes to provide relief to their community's destitute had to correspond to the obligation of the able-bodied poor to work. The role of poor 'overseers' was codified with the predominant function to 'set the poor to work', including children whose parents were incapable of performing labour activities.[12] In line with the existing legislative framework, the Elizabethan Acts also ordered that poor relief recipients who refused to work should be sent to the House of Correction, and even to jail.

The public preoccupation with the correction of the poor was not arrested by the Elizabethan solution of providing 'work for those that will labour, punishment for those that will not and bread for those that cannot' (Dunning, quoted in Eden, 1797: 225). It would be incorrect to think that the sole concern of the poor legislation was an economic one, namely that of transforming the 'idle poor into the industrious poor' (Dean, 1991: 35). Contemporaries were only too aware, in fact, of the castigating capacity of the different options available for the governance of the poor. As the problem of poverty became increasingly tackled by local administrations with the institution of public workhouses, the physical confinement of the poor began to be widely discussed (and in some cases opposed) as the best possible solution for maintaining and punishing the poor at the same time (Rose, 1805: 36).[13] A vast pamphlet literature produced in seventeenth- and early eighteenth-century England attests to such a discussion and to the great concern for the *discipline* of the poor. Indirectly, such a debate testifies to the understanding of poverty at that time as being predominantly caused by individual misconduct, if not criminal inclination.

Moved by the idea that 'regulation of the poor' and their behaviour was needed (Defoe, 1704: 70), a number of remedies against poverty and idleness were proposed, not only by politicians but also economists, philosophers, novelists and preachers. These solutions would range greatly: from the provision of 'in kind' benefits so as to correct the poor's dietary conduct (first and foremost their inclination to spend their money in 'ale houses and brandy shops') and the obligation to wear a badge on their clothing so as to 'keep them submissive and orderly' (Dunning, 1698: 50), to the enslavement of 'incorrigible rogues' (Alcock, 1752: 60). Furthermore, most of these proposals would view the increase in destitution and vagabondage as a direct consequence of 'the relaxation of discipline and the corruption of manners', as famously maintained by John Locke (1697: 184), and therefore simply conclude that the idle poor should be obligated to work. Locke himself advanced the idea of putting poor children above three years of age into 'working schools' so as to eliminate the cost of their parents' relief rate while, at the same time, initiating them into 'religion, morality' and 'industry' (ibid.: 454–455). The (failed) 'Speenhamland experiment' wage-supplementation system of 1795–1834 (Speizman, 1966; Paz-Fuchs, 2008: 88), with its 'generous' detrimental effects

(Polanyi, 1944 [1957]), contained all the traits of a tentative and awkward 'transition to a capitalist modernity' (Dean, 1991: 159). However, its introduction only added to growing concern about the 'new' problem of *pauperism* in England: the alleged *dependence* of the poor upon the relief system. 'Moral panic' (Cohen, 1972 [2002]: 1) about the figure of dependent, 'voluntary' paupers (Dunkling, 1982: 10) and their potential threat to society became rampant again in this period and sparked a new debate about the methods used for their 'management' (Rose, 1805).

More increasingly the case was put for a *behavioural* rather than merely economic solution to the spread of pauperism. At the same time, the need for a reconceptualisation of the very term 'labouring poor' and its 'foolish' use in politics was advanced (Burke, 1791: 519) on the grounds that a 'young healthy man' cannot be called 'poor'. Abolitionists simply saw pauperism as a 'social cancer' (Poynter, 1969: 295) and called for the immediate interruption of the preceding 'generous' approach to the undeserving poor.

This discussion culminated in a new, nationally unified 'body of criminal law' (Webb, 1928: 3) that formalised the moral argument against the able-bodied male adult as a distinctive category of 'undeserving' claimant who, in fact, even lost his right to be considered 'poor'. In practical terms, the Victorian Poor Law brought two new innovations: the quasi-elimination of relief for able-bodied individuals, which became *conditional* upon confinement in the workhouse; and the introduction of a work incentive mechanism known as *less eligibility*. In retrospect one can only look at the introduction in 1723 of the 'workhouse test' – i.e. only those in a *true* condition of need would accept the severe living conditions of the workhouse – as an important precursor to the forthcoming legal exclusion of the 'able-bodied indigent' (Castel, 2003: 4) from *outdoor relief* actions that came to be applied with the new system.

Profoundly inspired by the philosophical and political views of its 'spiritual fathers', Malthus and Bentham (Edsall, 1971: 2; see also Fraser, 1976; Dean, 1991), the Poor Law Amendment Act of 1834 was influenced by two fundamental ideas.[14] Firstly, and in accordance with Malthus' beliefs on the role played by the old Poor Laws in raising 'the price of provisions', reducing the real price of labour and weakening 'one of the strongest incentives to sobriety and industry' (Malthus, 1798 [1805: 411]), advocates of the new reform were convinced of the need to break with the 'dependence' of the able poor on the existing system. It is true that Malthus' appeal for the complete abolition of relief for able-bodied males and their families was not ultimately incorporated into the new legislation. However, the conditions under which the new Poor Law provided for this category (i.e. their physical internment in the workhouse) introduced the abolitionist's solution for all intents and purposes. The formal and stigmatising distinction in the treatment of deserving and undeserving claimants was undoubtedly somehow inspired by Malthus' very preoccupation with the public subsistence of the 'labouring poor' and the moral 'perfectibility of man' (1798: 34, 98). Secondly, the new poor law was largely inspired by Bentham's basic idea that 'Charity-maintenance [maintenance at the expense of others] should not be made *more desirable* than self-maintenance for paupers' (1796: 267, emphasis added).

Thus, if Malthus' legacy can be said to have delivered the argument for the 'indoor' confinement option for undeserving claimants (i.e. the workhouse), Bentham provided a 'practical' solution to the *work incentive* dilemma in his own and future societies: the less eligibility mechanism.[15] Together, these two innovations became successful instruments for achieving the four predominant objectives of the reform: *reducing the cost* of poor relief (Fitzpatrick et al., 2006); *discouraging idleness* (Crowther, 1981); *disciplining the poor*; and, most interestingly, *isolating* them so that they could not 'infect' the rest of society with their diseases, vice and immorality (Lees, 1998: 126–129). With such an exacerbation of the spatial confinement option for the undeserving poor, therefore, the workhouse system came to function as a comprehensive and coherent system for the management of the poor: not only a punishing instrument and isolating institution but also a place of moral correction, a proper 'educational machinery' that could 'shape popular behaviour' and efficiently deter poor people from preferring public relief to work (Wiener, 1990: 153; see also Newman, 2014). As Polanyi poignantly described the situation, 'hunger was a better *disciplinarian* than the magistrate' (1944: 120, emphasis added).

As was the case in other parts of Europe, the new English Poor Law was essentially the incoherent product of diverse and frequently opposing moral, political and economic arguments for or against poor relief. Such an ambiguity is best explained following Taylor's view that the new Victorian system was essentially a 'compromise' through which some departure from the *laissez-faire* was conceded in the domain of poor relief for the sake of 'public morality', but only as long as the workhouse test and the less eligibility mechanisms could guarantee that the 'able-bodied pauper was forced down to the meanest level of subsistence' (Taylor, 1972: 42, 45).

This kind of debate, and the constant search for economic and moral remedies against poverty and idleness, was not exclusive to the English context. Especially in the aftermath of the Industrial Revolution, most European countries had to face the explosion of misery and find new ways of dealing with its increasing visibility. However, while in England poor relief actions soon became almost the exclusive responsibility of (national and local) public policy, in Catholic countries anti-poverty interventions remained far more variegated, with private philanthropy, religious charity, mutual help and institutional assistance being four different but often overlapping components of an 'organised culture of charity' (Pullan, 1995: 9).

The Italian context provides the archetypal reference for this model. The history of poor relief actions in pre-unification Italy contains a rich inventory of experiments and social innovations designed to tackle urban misery (Geremek, 1994; Albini, 2002).[16] One might be tempted to assume that the long and variegated tradition of private and religious assistance in Italian cities played a certain role in *diluting* the public preoccupation with the discipline of the poor that in other countries, such as England and France, came to take the form of a true 'anxiety of idleness' from the sixteenth century onwards (Geremek, 1994; Jordan, 2003). In this regard, it is significant to find, among the above-mentioned social innovations, at least three different antecedents of the poor-houses. *Hospitalia, diaconiae* and *xenodochia* (the latter being a former term for the *hospitium pauperum*) were Catholic charitable facilities generally admini-strated by confraternities and established in Italy during the early Middle Ages with the main function of 'hosting' and providing shelter, food and medical assistance not only to the poor but also to vagrants, pilgrims and every man, woman or child in need of protection (Morini, 1995; Albini, 2002; Dey, 2008).[17]

Interestingly, while it is true that these institutions flourished almost every-where in Europe, in Italy they became increasingly more organised during the fifteenth century, and in fact took on the role as the principal providers of assistance to the poor (Bianchi and Słoń, 2006). The social function fulfilled by these facilities was not, however, exclusively that of assisting the needy. They would also and predominantly provide the opportunity of performing a moral obligation to help the poor. The use of religious and private forms of charity as a means of honouring a spiritual and public duty, but also a 'calculated devotion' (Albini, 2002: 56),[18] is pivotal in order to fully understand the 'pervasive influence' (Kazepov, 2015: 102) of the Catholic Church in Southern Europe and, in particular, its role in the formation of the Italian model of assistance to the poor, and its ambivalences.

On the one hand, it is undeniable that the multifaceted public function of religious institutions represented a major feature of the Italian approach to solidarity. It is commonly assumed that the organization and attitude of con-fraternities' charitable institutions encapsulated the very essence of the Catholic *caritas* and *hospitality*, of which the Benedictine rule that all guests, *especially the poor*, should be welcomed 'as Christ in person' is but one example.

On the other hand, it would be incorrect to assume that Italy was an exception to the overall climate of 'moral panic' around pauperism that dominated Europe during the sixteenth and seventeenth centuries, and to the general efforts of both secular and religious authorities to 'spatially' repress the poor, discipline them and set them to work. Among these efforts, the papal edict of 1561 against begging has been described as 'symptomatic' of a profound transformation in attitudes to poverty (Geremek, 1994: 212) and marks the beginning of a new era of social and spatial confinement of poverty in Catholic countries. Arguably, the adoption of this approach in Italy resulted in a further exacerbation of the ambivalent approach towards the poor. One of the best examples of the 'unease coexistence' (Pullan, 1976: 25) of two opposite attitudes regarding poverty in Italian culture (its sanctification and demonisation) is found in the 'triumphs of charity' in the sixteenth century: the local poor were 'publicly exhibited' in a parade during which they would accept almsgiving; under the eye of the town's populace, they would then be accompanied to the local hospital so as to 'underline the victory of public charity over the indecorous act of mendicancy' (Pullan, 1995: 9). As a result, the public stigmatisation of the poor and the community's compassion and sense of solidarity towards them would fuse. The rhetoric underlying these actions – that mendicants and beggars must be helped but only in such a way as to guarantee their separation from the 'respectable community' (Pullan, 1995) – became increasingly impassioned as public concern about the concentration of beggars in urban areas and the potential consequences for social order grew (Fatica, 1982).[19] In fact, this argument was thus gradually substituted by the case for the moral and disciplinary correction of the undeserving poor and their internment in dedicated hospices,[20] with the two-fold advantage of 'identifying the *truly* needy' (widows, orphans elderly people and the disabled) and eliminating the continuous pestering of many beggars in the streets (Muratori, 1723: 657).[21]

The erection of these buildings in Italy, more frequent after 1650, embodied this very rhetoric and the underlying shift from 'hospital care' to the 'disciplinary institute' as an architectural solution to the problem of pauperism – or at least to its potential disruptive impact on the urban, non-poor population. Significantly, however, both the semantic and architectural dimensions of the Italian hospices signal a profound contrast with the English workhouses. Whereas the 'moral architecture' of the English workhouses was essentially one of 'visual and aural' surveillance and institutional control of the inmates as well as a constant reminder to paupers of their powerless state as prisoners (Newman, 2013: 131–133), the Italian *alberghi dei poveri* – literally 'hotels for the poor' – were accurate reflections, at least in their aesthetics, of the exaltation of Catholic *caritas*.

Designed precisely *not* for the paupers but rather 'for their management', the 'moral geometry' (Driver, 1993: 3, 65) of most English workhouses[22] famously reproduced Bentham's ideas for his Panopticon (1778) and its underlying model in which the constant centralised surveillance of the inmates would lead to their 'moral health' (Bentham, 1796), as would the 'bareness and squalor' of certain premises, indicated by the Commission on the Poor Laws in 1909 (Driver, 1993: 6).

By contrast, a consistent evolution of the former 'triumphs' of charity and their public significance, the Italian counterparts of these institutions were architectural manifestations of the country's ambiguous sentiments and approach to poverty. The construction of the monumental *Albergo dei poveri* ('Palace of Mercy') in Genoa, is said to have been driven by the idea that it should have displayed 'the royal magnificence of Genoa's piety' so as to cause in the eye of the viewer the highest admiration for its generosity and charity'.[23] At the same time though, as was the case with the English workhouses (whose architecture was only functional to their controllers/administrators), the Italian *alberghi dei poveri* were not designed for their own paupers. In fact, the main aim of the architectural opulence of these buildings, as has been poignantly noted (Nicoloso, 1995), was to welcome the wealthy benefactors visiting the institutions. This is not to say that the 'magnificent' spatial reclusion of mendicants in Italian cities did not also serve disciplining and economic purposes. Quite the contrary in fact; and, in spite of the frequent lack of a central point of control and management in some of the Italian hospices (for example in Naples; see Guerra, 1995), these institutions attempted to perform the same reforming function as the English workhouse. All in all, it can be argued that the *alberghi* were nothing more than 'anti-chaos machineries' (Canciullo, 2010: 240) that conveniently provided affordable and flexible labour responding to local economic requirements (Ciuffetti, 2004).[24] Yet, a certain difference between the two systems can be postulated, with the English workhouse being distinctively oriented to exert some degree of social control over the *industriousness* of the idle poor, and its Italian equivalent pursuing predominantly a *redeeming* function over its inmates (Pullan, 1988), subjected to 'more or less painful and backbreaking labour and an endless round of sacred readings and devotional activity' (Pullan, 1976: 33).

As a conclusion to this chapter, it is possible to think again of the tremendous and multifaceted role exerted by morality as a dimension in the construction of poor relief actions in different contexts. Our cross-sectional journey across the history of deservedness as a constant component in most public approaches to poverty is only a first step in our exploration of the issue. However, it has shown that, despite contextual differences, idleness, deviance and discipline present three recurrent themes in the history of poverty relief, emerging especially in times of social and economic crisis and in conjunction with the search for social innovations to tackle poverty and other unwanted phenomena. Moreover, this discussion has provided us with some important preliminary insights into the two divergent routes taken by Italy and England, and into the different moral and social backgrounds informing their public reactions to poverty as a phenomenon, predominantly driven up to the late modern era, by the common objective of performing a function of 'moral enlightenment' (Foucault, 1977: 248) or 'moral improvement' (Frampton, 1979: 369) of those deemed undeserving of community support.

The role of morality in the construction of solidarity and poor relief actions, we have seen, is at least two-fold. While the implicit attribution of expected social characteristics attached to the poor (idleness, crime, social deviance, perversity) has frequently resulted in attempts at moralising and disciplining the poor, moral and ethical backgrounds informing public policy actions of poor 'regulation' have played a major role in the construction of diverse *worlds of solidarity* in different contexts. To be sure, we can conclude this chapter by underlining that the dimension of morality in poor relief and solidarity actions is generally conducive to the exacerbation of the social separation, both symbolic and substantial, of the poor and the non-poor population into two different categories. One of the most important elements of social discipline and moralisation, the 'categorisation' of the poor in the English workhouse in different classes, was an essential mechanism of social separation, submission and alienation of the undeserving poor. This is not to say that the disciplining intention(s) of poor laws in pre-modern and modern times served the objective of moralisation alone. Quite the contrary in fact, this chapter has illustrated that the moralising approach towards the poor population was frequently instrumental to the achievement of social order and productivity goals. This is signalled, among other things, by the fact that the non-poor obsession with idleness and the consequent exacerbation of hostility towards those undeserving of social support emerged especially in conjunction with, or in the aftermath of, 'social crises' (such as epidemics, food crises and wars) that alternatively would increase the urban *visibility* of pauperism or augment the economic need for inexpensive 'labouring hands'.

Notes

1 Contributions to the discussion from other disciplines include the vast literature produced by Robert E. Goodin (1985; Goodin 1988; Goodin et al., 1987; Schmidtz and Goodin, 1998; Goodin and Le Grand, 1999) on the moral justifications for welfare interventions and the role of poor relief actions as a form of collective social responsibility, which provides a fundamental theoretical key for understanding the moral background of public policy interventions for the poor from a *philosophical* point of view.

2 Various studies have contested Plutarch's view that Pericles' building schemes were used to tackle *widespread unemployment* and have suggested that in his description the biographer might have been influenced by the situation of his own times rather than having reported reality at times of Pericles. This scholarship concluded that Plutarch's labour shortage was more likely than unemployment as a rationale for those schemes, considering the pace of Athens' expanding economy at that time (Frost, 1964). However, others have noted that Plutarch's reference to the elimination of laziness as an objective of these programmes is also emphasised and therefore must have been found in his own sources.

3 Plutarch, *The Life of Pericles* (emphasis added). Complete English text available at http://penelope.uchicago.edu/Thayer/E/Roman/Texts/Plutarch/Lives/Pericles*.html.

4 Many authors acknowledged that the extension of participation in *cleruchies* to the lower classes was done by Athens to raise its citizens from a condition of poverty to 'modest affluence' (see, for example, Jones, 1952: 17–18). Plutarch, *Life of Pericles*.

5 Cicero, *De Officiis*, I, 42–45.

6 2 Thess., 3:10. Biblical quotes are from http://biblehub.com.

7 The indication of a moral obligation of Christians to help those in need in the Bible is generally discussed with reference to the passage 'The poor you will always have with you', Matthew 26:11.

8 35 Ed. 1 C. 1, emphasis added.

9 Historical accounts of the anti-vagrancy legislation noted that the number of 'masterless' men wandering about in England during the XVI century was not sufficient to justify such a hostility against them (Beier, 1974).

10 Author's translation from Italian.

11 43 Eliz. I c. 2.

12 Geremek (1994: 166) reports that these overseers were in existence since 1536.

13 That was exactly the case made by MP George Rose (1805: 37), who contended that the elimination of the workhouse would have been 'as economical as humane'.

14 In this regard both Edsall (1971) and Dean (1991) note that although Malthus and Bentham were not part of the Poor Law Commission, their ideas became at the very least influential to the proposals that N. Senior and E. Chadwick brought to the Commissioner's Report prepared for the new legislation.

15 The 'less eligibility' principle was designed as an incentive to remain in the labour market and to guarantee at the same time that the situation of the individual receiving social assistance 'shall not be made really or apparently so eligible as the situation of the independent labourer of the lowest class. ... Every penny bestowed, that tends to render the condition of the pauper more eligible than that of the independent labourer, is a bounty on indolence and vice' (Poor Law Commissioners' Report of 1834: II.1.8). As the workhouse test, the less eligibility mechanism also performed an 'assessment' of the condition of true need among the poor.

16 The variegation and fragmentation of poor relief actions is also a direct consequence of the Italian political and territorial configuration. Up until Italian political unification in 1861, poor relief actions were necessarily administrated at the municipal level (*comuni*) and there was no such thing as a statutory national legislation regulating assistance to the poor. In such a fragmented landscape, the 'levelling' role played at that time by religious confraternities and Papal ordinances in their governance of pauperism, as well as a certain 'competitiveness' (Pullan, 1995) and 'best practices' exchange among Italian cities (see, for example, the case of mendicants' reclusion in Fatica) should not be underestimated.

17 In some cases, as in the hospital of Santa Maria dei Battuti in Treviso, assistance to the indigent would also include educational subsidies for capable girls (D'Andrea, 2003).

18 The theme of a 'calculated donation' among merchants in Milan is fully reported in Albini, 2002.

19 Among these was the possible transformation of beggars into 'professional mendicants' (Fatica, 1982)

20 Documents from the time attest, in fact, to a variegated classification of the poor and their respective 'spaces' of internment. In Modena, for example, urban non-able-bodied poor would be authorised to beg; the sturdy urban adult poor would be sent to the mendicants' hospital or to the poor hospice or set to work for rich or noble families; poor strangers from the countryside would be banned and exiled (see Fatica, 1982).

21 Author's translation from Italian, emphasis added.

22 For a review of architectural and functional diversity among English workhouses see again Driver (1993) or Newman (2013).

23 Document of mid-sixteenth century quoted in Ciucci (1995: 7) author's translation.

24 The Albergo dei Poveri in Naples is a known example of the failure of these institutions that eventually culminated also in its aesthetic and organisational decadence (for a description see Farrell-Vinay, 1989).

3 The moral backgrounds of the welfare state

Individualism and solidarity in the British and Italian contexts

From repression to prevention

Chapter 2 discussed how poverty has long been understood as a phenomenon *predominantly* derived from individual misconduct. It can be argued that until the late modern period not only governments' but also intellectuals' views on poverty and its main determinants played a major role in generating profound public misconceptions regarding both the 'worthy' and 'unworthy' poor, if not open hostility towards them (Coats, 1958: 38; Coats, 1976; Dean, 1991). Polanyi correctly recognises the role of the scientific and political narrative in creating a distorted representation of poverty, lamenting that at the end of the eighteenth century 'the true nature of pauperism was still hidden from the minds of men' (1944: 114). Needless to say, the moralisation of poverty did not disappear from one day to the next, but underwent a long and gradual process of transformation in parallel both with the emergence of more 'modern' and scientific explanations of its causes and with the construction of welfare institutions in the majority of industrialised countries. It is significant in this regard that the very word 'unemployment' only appeared in the *Oxford English Dictionary* for the first time as late as 1888 (Burnett, 1994).

The recognition of unemployment as an *involuntary* phenomenon can be considered as the first but fundamental milestone in the departure from poverty paradigms based on the assumed association between indigence and laziness and in the recognition that it is the 'condition' of unemployment to be 'problematic, not the individuals affected by it' (Himmelfarb, 1991: 41). Opening up to new but still tentative opportunities to comprehend the complex and multifaceted causes of poverty, the (partial) 'impersonalisation' of unemployment has been an important theoretical and social precursor of reforms aimed at *regulating* the economic and industrial system rather than the moral 'character' of the poor.

Not incidentally, it is precisely in the aftermath of these events that we can identify the emergence of fundamental social innovations concerning poor relief actions, including the *discovery of prevention* as a means of fighting destitution (Webb, 1928: 16) and the gradual 'democratisation of compassion' which occurred through the extension of welfare payments to the (formerly undeserving) working poor (Himmelfarb, 1991: 4). As an effect of these dynamics, and in conjunction with the gradual expansion of income support schemes in industrialised countries, the idea of the alleged moral characteristics of the poor being the *main* cause for their condition came under scrutiny by intellectuals and social reformers. However, this chapter will show that moralising approaches to poverty and the poor did not disappear.

The present chapter will look again at two apparently different models of solidarity for the poor, the Italian and the British cases. This time we will examine if and how the *moralising discourse* regarding the poor changed during the transition of these countries from a 'framework of repression' (Webb, 1928) of poverty – under which poor relief for able-bodied adults was 'virtually unobtainable' (Williams, 1981: 6) – to a system of 'prevention' wherein unemployment support became institutionalised: the modern welfare state. Far from being unidirectional and coherent, this process has been characterised by the increasing role of intermediate actors of social support. Especially during the second half of the nineteenth century, private philanthropy and charitable institutions played a complementary function to the one exerted by official systems of relief in both countries (as in other industrialised nations). Moreover, in one form or another, their work and ideas paved the way for new understandings of poverty and for the institutionalisation of public solidarity towards certain categories among the poor. It is thus appropriate to consider this particular period as the immediate precursor of the 'embryonic welfare state' (Morlicchio et al., 2002: 256), and thus to examine what happened to the moralisation of the poor discourse when collective solidarity began to emerge as a 'social issue'.

It is worth noting before undertaking our examination of these two countries that comparative social policy studies generally describe the British and Italian welfare and social systems in terms of their profound differences rather than their possible similarities. Typically, Great Britain is said to encapsulate most of the ideal-typical characteristics of the *liberal* world of welfare regimes (Esping-Andersen, 1990), with its strong emphasis on *laissez-faire* ideology, residualism and marketisation (Taylor, 1972; Spicker, 2013a), while the Italian case is generally portrayed with the typical traits of the *Mediterranean* model of social protection: fragmentation, dualism, familialism/familism and a rudimentary approach to social assistance (Leibfried, 1993; Ferrera, 1996; Rhodes, 1997; Gough, 2001; Morlicchio et al., 2002; Matsaganis et al., 2003; Ferrera, 2005; Ascoli and Pavolini, 2015). These differences, most scholars agree, are not accidental but are in fact the specific result of diverse 'value structures' and 'social norms' that have profoundly affected the overall development of welfare institutions at different stages and over the years (Clasen and Clegg, 2007; Schmidt, 2001; Mau, 2003). As ideal-typical categorisations, however, the British and the Italian welfare systems are far from being perfect reproductions of their correspondent archetypes. Rather, their past and present configurations may be understood in terms of dynamic systems that change and adapt across time. Nonetheless, their classification in 'clusters' has inevitably nourished a number of myths. Among these is the pervasive belief that the current British model of social protection for the poor is a residualist one wherein the state only intervenes on a last-resort basis (Titmuss, 1974), and for which *self-reliance* is the first and most important channel of wellbeing. Such a belief has been, in fact, discredited. Recent research has evidenced, for example, that 'extensive and inclusive' forms of social assistance significantly help reduce poverty in Britain (Gough, 2001; Ranci and Migliavacca, 2015). In a similar way, the emphasis placed on the alleged 'communitarian' culture of solidarity attributed to the Italian familialistic social system has erroneously led to the inappropriate conclusion that there is no such thing in Italy as the individualisation of social risks, which is generally considered a prerogative of the Anglo-Saxon systems. Dispelling these myths, or at least putting them in an historical perspective, is the overall objective of this chapter. We will retrace the moral and social backgrounds of their contemporary systems of social protection by looking at their common – but not necessarily identical and unidirectional – pathways towards what Lees (1998) has termed the 'rejection of residualism' and the emergence of collective forms of responsibility to the poor.

From religion to eugenics: Victorian confusion at the turn of the century

It has been argued that the expansion of communitarian and voluntary initiatives of poverty alleviation and mutual help at the end of the nineteenth century qualifies the late Victorian period as being the golden age of philanthropy (Himmelfarb, 1991; Prochaska, 1988; Hilton et al., 2012).[1] However, this should be contextualised and understood as just one of the manifold reactions of the English public to a new case of 'moral panic' at the end of the century: the urban *invasion* of the 'dangerous poor' (Morris, 2002).

Jones (1971: 224) poignantly described the emergence of an urban *degeneration* argument among the English middle classes as the culmination of increasing 'moral anxiety' and 'political fear' created by prolonged cyclical depression, labour market dynamics (among which the misunderstood role of casual and seasonal labour) and the onset of a housing crisis in London.[2] The degeneration theory, he points out, was the first step in the recognition of the potential effects of the environment on the individual, but did not eliminate the disciplining approach towards the poor who, in fact, became the subject of a new wave of moralisation when concern for the potential imminent unrest of the working class grew.

Charitable institutions were not alien to these transformations. Commentators have differed however on the role of civic and charitable movements in late Victorian England. Some, such as Gerturde Himmelfarb (1991: 384), maintain that the proliferation of these associations is *at least* indicative of the great effort and 'moral imagination' of social reformers, activists and academics of that time to find new solutions to social and moral problems such as destitution. Seen from this perspective, the philanthropic commitment of late

Victorians had a prominent role in paving the way for the 'demoralisation' of poverty and in the gradual shift to the collectivist solution to poverty: the welfare state. Others, such as Finlayson (1994: 91), advance the idea that a 'mutual reinforcement' of voluntarism and state interventions existed during the Victorian period, 'characterized by a common dislike of indiscriminate relief' seen as potentially conducive to pauperism. To be sure, the expansion of voluntary organisations dedicated to social problems testifies to an interesting phenomenon: the transformation of the religious and spiritual fervour of the late Victorians into a new religion of humanitarian 'compassion' (Himmelfarb, 1991) or even a 'secular faith' (Page, 1996: 40), in some cases accompanied by the increasing reliance on a new, 'scientific' approach to social issues. It is not incidental that two of the first scientific attempts at measuring poverty appeared precisely in this period. Charles Booth's monumental survey (*The Life and Labour of People of London*, 1889–1903), often considered the 'starting point of all serious discussion' of poverty (Englander, 1998: 59), proved to the public that poverty could be counted and mapped, while Seebohm Rowntree (1901) offered the first measurement of the phenomenon based on the use of a 'poverty line'.[3]

Humanitarianism and liberalism, however, were not the predominant, let alone the sole, ideological roots of the Victorian approach to poverty. The new *positive* philosophy, with its emphasis on scientific (rather than theological) knowledge as a method of understanding and changing reality is one important factor in the emergence of a tentatively more 'humanitarian' attitude towards poverty. Positivist ideas envisaged the advent of a 'religion […] without a God', to quote John Stuart Mill (1865: 39), wherein 'obligations of duty [and] sentiments of devotion [are addressed] to a concrete object … the Human Race'.

Famously, positivism also postulated the reconciliation of moral and social *order* with scientific *progress* (Comte, 1851; see also Lenzer, 1975: 502–503), thus attracting and at the same time *confusing* the English middle classes (Harp, 1995).[4] At the same time, Social Darwinism and the application of the 'struggle for existence' argument (Darwin, 1859 [2005]: 60) to the social world added a biological perspective in support of the urban degeneration thesis. By advancing the idea of a progressive 'hereditary deterioration' of the urban poor (Jones, 1971: 287; Morris, 2002) Social Darwinism also consigned to the British middle classes a 'natural' explanation for their anxieties of *fin-de-siècle* (Ledger, 1995) and a justification for their paternalistic attitude towards the poor.

As a consequence of such a broad-ranging discussion, philanthropic organisations did not share a common vision in their treatment of poverty. In fact, even within the domain of civic institutions acting in this period, the distinction is usually drawn between their different attitudes. In particular, and interestingly, it is precisely these organisations and their different ideas that one can look at to discuss the slow departure of late Victorians from their own 'obsession' with morality (Himmelfarb, 1991: 7).

One of the most active and discussed philanthropic associations, the Charity Organisation Society (CSO) – founded in 1869 under the name the Society for Organising Charitable Relief and Repressing Mendicity – for example, has been frequently criticised as the personification of what remained of Britain's hostile and moralising attitude that inspired the Poor Laws. In an attempt at reconciling Christian *caritas* and the evangelisation of the poor (Brundage, 2002) with the modern Malthusian doctrine (Lewis, 1995: 27) and a scientific approach to pauperism, the CSO produced a strategy for poverty relief which was 'paradoxical' to say the very least (Searle, 1998: 192). Influenced by positivism and Social Darwinism alike, the CSO not only promoted the idea that 'scientific investigations' could help identify the *truly* deserving cases and discipline the undeserving ones (Whelan, 2001). It also introduced, via the ideas of one member and activist Helen Dendy, a new *bio-moral* categorisation of poor deservedness based on the distinction between the 'true industrials' and the 'residuum', the latter being characterised by the lack of any 'economic virtues', 'a low order of intellect, and a degradation of the natural affections to something little better than animal instincts' (Dendy, 1893: 601). Dendy's ideas, whether corroborated or inspired by Charles Booth's (1903) similar conclusions on the demoralised character of a small part of London's population – and its required urban segregation – gave life to a true *residuum frenzy* among Victorian movements at the turn of century which culminated in a eugenic deviation:[5] inheritance and transmission of blastophthoria – the degeneration of the germ cells believed to be due to chronic poisoning (namely, alcohol) – among the urban poor became an accepted reinterpretation of pauperism and the subject of scientific research by the Eugenic Society (Freeden, 1979; Mazumdar, 1980; Paul, 1984; Leonard, 2005).

Commentaries on the CSO approach have generally expressed a strong criticism for its 'anachronistic' (Jones, 1971: 313) concern for the urban repression of poverty and mendicancy (derived from a misunderstanding of the new industrial society and its economic problems); the rejection of indiscriminate almsgiving; and the insistence on self-reliance and behavioural treatments of undeserving cases. As such, the CSO has been generally described as the last bulwark of Victorian individualism and *laissez-faire* (Mowat, 1961; Roof, 1972; Rose, 1972; Finlayson, 1994; Humphreys, 2001). An example of the CSO's moralising attitude towards those claiming support is its very 'invention' of *home visits* as an instrument for caseworkers to derive 'a narrative of moral character, deservingness and *helpability* from the scattered objects of the life of the poor' (Livesey, 2004: 55, emphasis added).[6]

The CSO's role in the perpetuation of an old 'individualistic' and moralising approach to poverty is often contrasted with the collectivist 'spirit' of the Fabian Society (Roof, 1957: 20). Although it was not a 'provider' of charitable care, activists from the Fabian movement were strong advocates of a *political* resolution of poverty. Profoundly inspired by the socialist reforming views of two of its most prominent members, Sidney and Beatrice Webb, it strongly opposed the Poor Law system and made the case for a much more extensive state intervention.

The reform proposals delivered by CSO and the Fabian activists at the Royal Commission on the Poor Laws (1905–1910) have been described, until very recently, as the epitome of these two apparently contrasting visions, led by the two most prominent frameworks of the time: *laissez-faire* and interventionism (Fraser, 1973). The resulting *Majority Report* (expression of the CSO's values) presented the problem of poverty as essentially a matter of moral failure and encouraged self-help individualism and the continuation of the workhouse system (Bosanquet, 1910), while the *Minority Report* (behind which the main force was Beatrice Webb) insisted on the social and economic need to 'break up with the Poor Law' and eliminate the workhouse. Contemporary studies, however, have downplayed the apparent contrasting positions of the CSO and the Fabian Society (Himmelfarb, 1991; Vincent, 1984; Englander, 1998). These accounts have correctly evidenced that mid- to late Victorian reformers and commentators from both parties still had a 'moral mind' when the problem of poverty was taken into account. Both Fabian and CSO activists, like the majority of their contemporaries, had no 'real conception' of the labour market and its principal dynamics, and would generally misinterpret unemployment, casual labour and poverty as expressions of a 'demoralisation' of the character (Jones, 1971: 262; see also Webb, 1909).

By and large, it can be argued, the social background of solidarity and poor relief at the end of the nineteenth century was still predominantly based on the assumption that excessive doles could 'corrupt' the character of the recipient. While calling for the increased preventive role of the state, Beatrice and Sidney Webb themselves strongly opposed the idea of a universal and compulsory insurance against sickness on the grounds that it would have been tantamount to the government 'paying the people to be ill' (Webb and Webb, 1911: 186). With their conflicting, but not necessarily irreconcilable, visions for the future of the poor relief system, in fact, the CSO and the Fabian Society were a product of their times, with the growing uncertainty and anxiety regarding the future combined with an irreducible fascination with the new positive philosophy. The very fact that even socialist reformers Sidney and Beatrice Webb were somehow attracted by the argument of 'congenital defects' as a cause of urban pauperism is indicative of the confusion regarding the social, moral, economic and biological interpretations of poverty at the turn of the century. While expressing some scepticism of the Eugenic Society's views on poverty, the Webbs failed to resist the lure of evolutionist and Malthusian interpretations of pauperism alike.[7] They made an explicit case for a eugenic 'revolution' and enthusiastically commented that, under the Poor Laws system, '*it is exactly [the idle and the thriftless, the drunken and the profligate] and practically these only, who at present make full use of their reproductive powers*', thus alimenting 'the reproduction of mental, moral and physical defectives' (Webb and Webb, 1911: 240, original emphasis). Regardless of these interpretations however, both the role of Fabianism and that of the CSO are recognised today as important precursors to the establishment of the modern British welfare state. We can agree in this regard with Himmelfarb

(1991: 385) that the social reform movements of this period, with their diverse and often incoherent efforts to deal with the problem of poverty, are the personification of the late Victorian age as an 'interregnum between the past and the present' that however managed to lead British society towards the establishment of its contemporary welfare state.

The slow emergence of 'disinterested morality' in Italy

In Italy, the discourse on poverty as a social question has emerged relatively recently, at least from an *institutional* point of view. Relief of poverty, as we saw in Chapter 2, was by no means unacknowledged in late-modern Italy, but it was mainly tackled as either a matter of *urban emergency* (and treated with the physical confinement of the poor in working/disciplining institutions) or as a 'moral' and collective duty left to the voluntary agency of private and religious charity. In spite of the long recognition, in the tradition of Catholic countries, of a moral obligation to help the poor, it was Italy that perhaps struggled the most to accept the public role of the state in relieving destitution or, in short, to incorporate a 'disinterested morality' of help and support for the poor into its legal system.

While in other contexts, and most notably in England, poor relief became the subject of public debate and statutory national legislation as early as the beginning of the seventeenth century, in Italy a proper national debate on this matter only came about after its political unification in 1861. However, and despite this significant difference, the Italian context of the late nineteenth century was not entirely dissimilar from the English one as both countries remained strongly dependent on the role of private and voluntary philanthropy for the relief of their poor, with most of the legislation only dedicated to suppressing mendicity and vagabondage. Even before Italian political unification, which is generally regarded as the major watershed in the introduction of a national political debate on poverty, at least 25 different *categories* of philanthropic organisations devoted to relief of the poor could be enumerated (Fiori, 2005), most of them administered by the Catholic Church. The emergence of a collective concern for the relief of poverty in Italy, however, is by no means comparable with the activism of the Victorian middle classes. It would be tempting to postulate that the phenomenon of poverty was much less visible and urgent as a social and political issue in Italy (as compared to England and other countries) as a result of its delayed industrialisation and lower levels of urbanisation (Malanima, 2005), but in reality urban and rural poverty was as visible in Italy as in other European regions, and recurrently even more pressing a social problem when labour market crises erupted.

Thus, the political and intellectual elites of the new United Kingdom of Italy did express their interest in researching and eliminating the real causes of destitution,[8] but the reform process followed an ambiguous path. On the one hand, the introduction of the new Italian penal code in 1889 marked some departure from the penal punishment of 'suspicious persons' – a category that would include 'idle persons, vagabonds and mendicants'[9] – and its substitution with a more 'progressive' legislative framework for the treatment of this group,[10] while on the other hand, public security and emergency laws maintained a *repressive* and policing apparatus for the 'dangerous' classes, a remnant of Napoleonic rule in Italy. Most studies agree today that the resulting system was only apparently contradictory. Aiming at guaranteeing that public freedom would not benefit people with 'criminal intentions' – i.e. the 'dangerous classes' (Bolis, 1871: 183) – the general penal framework would stand as a safeguard to liberal rights, leaving to the police and the administration the task of defending the social order from potential threats (Da Passano, 2004).

This *modus operandi* was also consistent with the general approach to the problem of poverty of this period, centred on the repression of economically dangerous individuals, the idea being that charitable almsgiving would provide for others. Reliance on the voluntary work of Catholic charities as the predominant channel for relieving the needy became institutionalised in 1862, when a law was passed giving autonomy to these institutions – called *Opere Pie* – in their philanthropic activities. We could draw an analogy with the Italian complementary role of state actions (dedicated to repressing/punishing mendicancy and setting the poor to work) and voluntary charitable relief with the Poor Law system that existed in Britain during the same period. Yet, two important distinctions should be made in this regard. Firstly, and unlike their Victorian counterparts, Italian charities at the mid–end of the century were still predominantly administered by Catholic institutions with the main objectives of providing for the 'moral and material' relief of the poor and, at the same time, encouraging religious education (Scaglia, 1863: 23). Secondly, in the absence of any *formalisation* of public commitment against destitution, the very identification of undeserving categories of poor remained, to say the least, much vaguer in its application in the Italian context compared to the English case, and predominantly applied to those considered to be 'false poor'.

This is not to say that there was no such thing in Italy as an attempt at providing 'scientific' explanations and methods to the problem of poverty and its 'demoralising' effect on the individual. Philanthropist Baron de Gérando's book *Le visiteur du pauvre* appeared in France in 1820, advancing the idea that 'visiting the poor', observing them in person and repeatedly 'ascertaining' their true condition of need and their 'moral history' of idleness (1832: 48–49) was the only viable method for *targeting,* as we would say today, 'true indigents' and providing them with charitable help. Frequently regarded as an advocate of the deserving/undeserving poor separation and its rationalisation, de Gérando's work was in reality a strong critique of Malthusianism and contained a much more modern vision of poor relief than one might think: that a 'sublime' form of 'disinterested morality' should govern the rich–poor relationship and that humanity should act as a whole 'family' (ibid.: 37). Unlike Britain, where de Gérando's views had apparently little resonance, Italian reformers were somehow receptive to his ideas, and especially to the possibility he offered to 'accommodate Christian charity and economic progress through adminis-trative action' (Woolf, 1991: 58). Economist Petitti di Roreto was probably the most influenced by the work of de Gérando, who was applauded in the former's famous treatise on mendicancy and charity (1837) but rejected at the same time for his method of 'visiting the poor', considered simply impractic-able. While he posited that '*all* true mendicants need and have the right to receive support', Petitti specified that the different categories of beggars should be treated differently:

- work for the able-bodied (via internment in the workhouse);
- shelter and support for the non-able poor;
- charity for the 'shameful' poor;
- detention for the 'supposed' poor, i.e. the 'true scroungers' of society (1837: 29, 31).[11]

Petitti's treatise was not morality free. It was certainly imbued with both Christian values and paternalistic views on the role that 'religion and humanity' should play together to 'temper and correct' the 'moral disease' of pauperism (ibid.: 120). At the same time, however, his work was a forerunner in its plea for *public relief* to the poor and in its discussion of an Italian 'taboo': the substitution of religious and spontaneous almsgiving with what was referred to as 'legal charity'.

This and other treatises attest to the existence of a debate on the legalisation of charity, but nonetheless Italy proved resistant to change. By the end of the nineteenth century, there was no sign of the complex system used in England to 'scientifically' test deservedness and distinguish between different categories of needy. One could assume that Petitti and de Gérando's scientific methods were way more challenging in their concrete *application* because Italian charity was imbued with a pronounced 'humanitarianism', derived from its Catholic nature (Woolf, 1991: 62); but, in fact, both Catholic and non-religious reformers and commentators expressed their concerns about the elimination of 'false' pauperism from the Italian streets (see, for example, Morichini, 1870). Nevertheless, such a concern was rarely put into action.[12] Political instability and fragmentation, on the other hand, proved much more powerful than religion in obstructing, or at least procrastinating social reforms (Farrell-Vinay, 1989). As a consequence of the Italian reluctance to reform its system, the state's approach to charity for the poor remained by and large unchanged until the end of the century. Professional beggars would be the most and probably the only 'suspicious' category to be formally excluded from charity support, while discretionary selectivity remained the rule of thumb when it came to voluntary charity.

The belated emergence of a public national debate on the treatment of poverty in Italy and the lack of coordination among the numerous philan-thropic organisations active in the Peninsula must of course be considered important factors in the delayed formalisation of 'eligibility' in relief actions.

It is a fact, however, that a strong political resistance existed to the very idea of regulating charity and making it 'legal'. The *laissez-faire* approach of early Italian governments to the problem of poverty is generally interpreted as inspired by the liberal views of the Historical Right (*Destra Storica*). In reality though, liberal views on the role of private charity as the ideal instrument of poverty relief were common to left- and right-wing exponents alike, who would look with scepticism at the prospective elimination of Catholic almsgiving. They feared the English example and often evoked the 'ghost of pauperism' and its vicious cycle, criticised by statesman Count Camillo Cavour himself:[13] the argument was that it was precisely the suppression of religious orders in England that had *produced* pauperism and consequently urged the creation of its expensive system of public relief. Still in 1880 Silvio Spaventa, one of the most prominent spokesmen of the Historical Right and fiery opponent of any alteration to the status quo in the domain of charity, made a very clear case against the transformation of the existing system into the 'legalisation' of charity (Camera dei Deputati, 1913):[14]

> Two different systems of charity exist. The first one, which is just like ours, relies upon natural instinct, human benevolence of individuals alone or associated. The State only intervenes to regulate such a benevolent instinct [...] but nothing more than that. It does not burden the taxpayers to supply this kind of support. The second system is based on the obligation of the State to help the poor. This is not our own and I hope it will never be.[15]

It is thus unsurprising that the Italian state only assumed a 'regulatory responsibility' for social welfare for the first time in 1890 (Borzaga, 2004: 51), when Prime Minister and exponent of the Historical Left Francesco Crispi broke the 'dogma' (Farrell-Vinay, 1989: 366) and signed a new law regulating the transformation of *Opere Pie* into '(quasi) public' institutions (Ranci, 1994: 251). Whereas the law was a further acknowledgement of the pivotal role of private charity in supporting and caring for the needy, it has also been seen, in retrospect, as the product of a new 'vision' of a forthcoming model of public aid (Silvano, 2007: 31). An apparently 'irrational rationalisation' of the system, the Crispi law was not only a feasible political solution that interrupted Italian inertia; it was also, in the view of many commentators, a 'flexible' instrument to adapt a national law to an extremely fragmented and inhomogeneous country in terms of labour market dynamics, industrialisation and urbanisation levels (Farrell-Vinay, 1989).

As was the case in Britain (and in other European countries), the turn of the century for Italy was a time of compromise between old moralising remnants of the past and utopian (or at least more progressive) views for the future. This affected not only the political visions of the elites but also the intellectual community and the poverty epistemology. As elsewhere in Europe, Italian scholarship was fascinated by the new evolutionistic explanations of society offered by biology, positivism and Social Darwinism. However, this affected the Italian production of 'scientific' knowledge regarding poverty and its causes in a distinctive manner. On the one hand, eugenics and the theory of degeneration became very popular among Italian socialists, as was the case in Britain. However, while the Webbs came to believe in a Malthusian interpretation of pauperism and made the argument for 'congenital defects', their own Italian socialists took a different approach and attributed the degeneration and demoralisation of the proletariat to social and economic causes: first and foremost, the exploitation of the working class by the economic elites. From this perspective, poverty and degeneration were not inherited and transmitted from generation to generation, as British and French eugenicists contended, but were a product of the capitalist society (Gervasoni, 1997).

On the other hand, the application of evolutionist theories to social issues such as poverty assumed a very dark tone in Italy when it offered a scientific justification for 'eugenic interventionism' (see Cassata, 2011 for a discussion). Not only, as in other countries, did the degeneration theory provide new grounds for the criminalisation and stigmatisation of the urban and rural poor alike as deviant, 'inferior' individuals, as anthropologist Niceforo claimed (1908: 68). The literature produced by a number of Italian exponents of the Lombrosian and eugenic school – such as anthropologist Giuseppe Sergi and, later, statistician Corrado Gini – also created a scientific legitimisation for experiments of social eugenics of which the totalitarian projects of the 'betterment of race' and 'racial hygiene' are only too infamous.

Was it the end of the moralisation of poverty? It might be true that traditional explanations of poverty in terms of morality did lose some ground in both Italy and Britain at the end of the century. However, they were replaced by eugenic, evolutionist and even racial interpretations that, under the guise of new 'scientific' paradigms, perpetuated and dangerously validated old doctrines and 'moral' prejudices against the poor – their assumed 'mental' and physical inferiority, deviance, dissolute behaviours and even genetic defects. How this was different in any meaningful way from the moralising and punishing attitudes towards the 'unworthy' immoral paupers of late modernity is hard to say. To be sure, whether explicitly referred to or implied by means of scientific paradigms, the moralisation of poverty was far from dead.

Welfare states and morality: break or continuity?

So far, we have discussed the social and cultural backgrounds of different systems of solidarity and poverty relief. In reality though, it is clear that the history of poor relief and the treatment of poverty until the beginning of the twentieth century is essentially the history of the moral and cultural backgrounds of political and intellectual elites deciding on the future of their poor populaces. Before the emergence of universal suffrage, decisions concerning the poor – and socio-economic rights in general – had little political resonance since people would have no instruments with which to 'sanction' these decisions in electoral terms. Politicians, at the same time, would not have specific mandates constraining their political operations. There was, of course, the possibility of social unrest, if not revolution – a constant menace in the case of unpopular decisions and, for many commentators, the real cause behind the 'invention' of the welfare state in Europe as a 'concession' made to the proletariat against the risk of communist insurrection and the revolutionary organisation of the working class (Flora and Heidenheimer, 1976).

In this regard, we can look at the events that occurred during the first half of the twentieth century as pivotal elements marking the transition to a new political emphasis on poverty as a collective problem. In 1908, the British Parliament approved the *Old Age Pension Act*, followed by the *National Insurance Act* in 1911. By including coverage for old age, sickness and unemployment (the latter restricted only to a part of the workforce), these Acts were the first steps in the recognition of a new understanding of poverty.[16] Most notably they acknowledged that poverty is profoundly linked to an individual's *life-cycle* and to income variation at different stages of one's existence, as advanced by Rowntree (1901), and that casual employment and under-employment produce *economic insecurity* even among those who are willing to work, as evidenced by one of the main designers of the National Insurance Act, William Beveridge.

The transposition of such a new knowledge framework around poverty into the public sphere is self-evident, for old age, sickness and unemployment became recognised 'risks' against which the population gained a statutory 'right' to be covered (Marshall, 1950). In 1919, Italy also introduced its first national insurance against old age and invalidity. Moreover, along with Great Britain it was one of the first countries to bring in unemployment insurance. How these and the following events led to the emergence of the modern welfare state in most European countries and under the pressure of what political, intellectual and historical circumstances this happened falls beyond the remit of this chapter. Whether it had its origins in a true sentiment of altruism and solidarity or as a new instrument designed to preserve the status quo (Baldwin, 1990), the introduction of preventive schemes of social security inaugurated a new era that culminated in the expansion of social security programmes during the *Trente Glorieuses* (1945–1975), the golden age of the Keynesian welfare state. Although social security schemes never included the entire population and public relief actions for the undeserving poor remained punitive in nature and residual in their extent, the emergence of the welfare state should not be underestimated in its effects on the de-moralisation of poverty.

For advocates of the 'liberal break' theory (Rimlinger, 1961; Flora and Heidenheimer, 1976) the new era initiated precisely with the introduction of national insurance, marking the 'breakthrough' of European welfare states in their departure from liberal ideas 'concerning the assignment of guilt and responsibility among the individuals, groups and the state'. The most radical break, their argument continues, occurred with the introduction of unemployment insurance that interrupted the underlying political resistance of previous political elites to supporting the clearest category of 'undeserving poor': non-working able-bodied individuals (Flora and Heidenheimer, 1976: 50, 51–52). The expansion of social security institutions is therefore a fundamental historical step for the gradual decline of moral and degrading classifications of the poor. The most important role of *contributory* insurance and social rights in this regard is that they diminished, albeit only temporarily, the idea of poor relief as being paid out of society's pockets and that of the poor as a 'public burden'. Further *specialisation* of preventive tools of social policy, with income support schemes increasingly designed to help distinct categories of the population (lone mothers, young adults, children, the long-term unemployed, etc.) was an additional element in this process. Eligibility rules paved the way for the *bureaucratisation of deservedness*: only those belonging to a certain category became eligible to receive support. Evidently, decisions concerning *what* categories among the poor are deserving of help, *how much* should they receive and under what *conditions* remained (and remains) a matter of moral and ideological perspective, as we will see in the following chapters. However, it is important to acknowledge at this point that the emergence of preventive schemes of social security at this stage of the welfare state's development reduced to some extent the *stigmatising* dimension of anti-poverty measures based on spatial reclusion, means-testing, home visits and behaviour tests for both deserving and undeserving poor.

The break with liberal approaches to solidarity, however, occurred at different speeds and in different ways in every country. In Britain, the construction of welfare institutions is said to have been distinctively influenced by new sentiments of collectivism and solidarity that emerged during the two world wars and in conjunction with the Great Depression of the 1930s (Titmuss, 1950). According to this line of interpretation, the wars had a major role in preparing the social and economic grounds for the expansion of the welfare state in the second half of the century (Page, 1996). The literature is divided however on the role of the *Beveridge Report* (1942) that famously established the basis for the new social contract. For many, William Beveridge, former research assistant of Beatrice Webb, is the indisputable *father* of the post-1945 egalitarian, universalistic, contributory social security system, and the very first advocate of the role of the welfare state in protecting the whole population against the famous 'Five Great Evils' of 'Want, Disease, Idleness, Ignorance and Squalor' (Hemerijck, 2013). Others remark that while it is true that the Beveridge Plan eliminated the bulk of means-tested benefits (Deacon and Bradshaw, 1983), it did not eliminate the less-eligibility principle (Veit-Wilson, 1992). Beveridge's safety net was, in fact, conceived to work (and could only work) under the assumption of a (quasi) full-employment situation, and predominantly for *insiders* of the system. The need to provide for proper anti-poverty instruments was overlooked as unnecessary, leaving only residual and means-tested social assistance to relieve the conditions of the 'true' outsiders. Women, an aspect much discussed by the feminist critique, only appeared in this system as mere 'accessories' to the male breadwinner and as part of a system designed to 'reinforce the values of a patriarchal, capitalist society' (Colwill, 1994: 54; see also Lister, 1990).

From this point of view, the Beveridge Plan has been interpreted not as a break with but in terms of a *continuity* with the liberal past. His residualist approach to the problem of 'want' – which paved the way for the institutionalisation of means-tested social assistance in the subsequent decades (Abel-Smith, 1992) – was not simply a reflection of an optimistic reliance on the new economic and social security system; it was also a vestige of the Victorian belief that the undeserving poor should rely first and foremost on self-help and charity for their subsistence (Harris, 1990). All in all, these accounts maintain that conditional and less eligible measures of relief continued to function as an instrument to exert social control over the poor population (Dominelli, 1988; Smith, 1997). In a similar albeit different vein, Jones and Novak (1999: 12) advanced the idea that a 'disciplinary' approach in poor relief actions can be looked at as the main characteristic of the British and other European welfare states during recent decades, of which the post-war 'social democratic' experience was only a brief departure from the 'coercive' approach generally used to discipline the poor in our society.

The development of the Italian welfare state in the post-war context differs profoundly from the British one, and not only for the diverse economic conditions in which Italy found itself in the aftermath of the First World War. The advent of fascism interrupted the new age of social reform initiated with the introduction of compulsory social insurance in 1919 (Ferrera, 1984). When the process of reform was restarted in the mid-1920s, it became an integral part of the totalitarian regime's ideology and its economic, political and social agenda. Three main and interlinked aspects can be said to have profoundly affected the future of the Italian welfare state and its overall approaches to poor relief and solidarity.

Firstly, there was Mussolini's 'obsession' with declining fertility rates in Italy. Famously, in his attempt at inverting the negative trend by means of maternity policies, Mussolini was not only driven by military and economic concerns but also by his aspirations of 'social hygiene' and what can be referred to as the moral 'regeneration' of the Italian populace (Quine, 2002). Eugenic concerns for the preservation of the Italian 'race' mixed with the pro-natalist exaltation of the family as a 'state institution' set the framework for the increasing social control of the state over the regulation of gender roles, with women 'elected' to perform predominantly reproductive and caring roles (Saraceno, 1991; de Grazia, 1992; Naldini, 2004). This element is frequently said to have had a tremendous 'cultural' effect on the successive development of the Italian welfare state in terms of social expectations on the part of the women and family in general. Most scholars in fact consider the fascist approach to the family as a core aspect in the subsequent 'familialisation of social assistance' in Italy (Saraceno, 1990; Saraceno, 1994).[17] Secondly, Mussolini's adversity to 'industrial urbanisation'[18] and his preference for the repression of urban poverty further procrastinated the debate on poverty and the identification of a national, institutional response to the increasing problem of destitution. Thirdly, the dramatic bureaucratisation of the regime's welfare apparatus, working as its 'consensus' machine, became a breeding ground for the eruption of cliente-listic exchanges (Ferrera, 1984: Ferrera, 1997), a major feature of the Italian post-war model of social protection (Saraceno and Negri, 1994; Ferrera, 1996). As is the case for Britain, a mix of continuity with the past and a break with the previous approach to poverty relief and solidarity is characteristic of the Italian embryonic welfare state and its successive phases of development. Other similarities between Italy and Britain lie in the *cultural assumptions* underlying the emerging welfare state in the post-war context. Among these assumptions, those regarding gender roles had, in both countries, a major role in characterising women as 'dependants' and in relegating them to reproducing and caring activities.

Compared to the British case it is more challenging, however, to detect the fundaments of the post-war Italian approach to poverty and social inclusion in the absence of a statutory social safety net for the poor. To be sure, it is precisely the overall *absence*, once again, of a proper debate on poverty and its elimination (which would be the subject of the first official national com-mission of inquiry only in 1951)[19] which was the recurrent theme of the Italian history of anti-poverty programmes, at least until very recently.

Notes

1 Friendly Societies are perhaps the best-known example of mutual help organisa-tions. Acting as both 'moral communities' (Weinbren and James, 2005: 100) and spaces of *reciprocity*, they performed the fundamental role of a *social safety net* for those in a situation of economic crisis that has been recognised only recently (Gorsky, 1998a; Gorsky, 1998b). Although a fundamental aspect of our discussion, Friendly Societies were predominantly instruments of social protections designed to secure the maintenance 'of the laborious poor' (Rose, 1805: 38). Society's true outsiders, most notably the (undeserving) very poor (who could not pay their membership fees) were substantially excluded from these organised forms of self-help.

2 Developed in the psychiatry domain at the end of the nineteenth century, the degeneration theory postulated the existence of an inherited 'pathological state' whose main symptoms would be 'crime, insanity, alcoholism, prostitution, vagrancy, suicide, and a number of organic disorders such as tuberculosis and syphilis' (see Nye, 1985: 663–664).

3 Rowntree (1901: 142) made a clear distinction between 'primary' and 'secondary' poverty: the latter included 'drinking, betting and gambling, [...] ignorant or careless housekeeping, and other improvident expenditures'.

4 Harp (1995: 36) postulated that 'its mixture of piety and science, atheism and morality and conservatism and social reform' allowed Victorians to legitimise 'science without destroying religious fervour or traditional morality'.

5 According to its founder, Francis Galton (1904: 1), eugenics is 'the science which deals with all influences that improve the inborn qualities of a race; also with those that develop them to the utmost advantage'..

6 It is uncertain whether the CSO and its designers were familiar with Baron de Gérando's work, *Le visiteur du pauvre*, which appeared in France in 1820 and was translated into English in 1832.

7 'There is no reason why those who are eliminated in the struggle of unrestricted competition should coincide with those whom we deem the unfit.' Beatrice Webb,

excerpt from An extended précis of a lecture delivered to the Eugenics Society at Denison House, Vauxhall Bridge Road, London on 15 December 1909.

8 This was urged, for example, during the Seventh Conference of Italian Scientists in Naples, 1845. See *Atti della settima adunanza degli scienziati italiani tenuta in Napoli*, Naples, 1846.

9 Codice Penale di S. M. il Re Di Sardegna Esteso Alle Due Sicilie, 1861.

10 Interestingly, while the new code eliminated idlers from the suspect categories, suspicion towards mendicants, and especially professional ones – referred to as *accattoni* – remained. Yet such a suspicion was reformulated in 'economic' terms. The new Zanardelli penal code prescribed detention for 'mendicants found possessing economic resources or objects *inappropriate* for their status whose origin could not be justified' (art. 492, Cod. Zanardelli).

11 Petitti also advocated a 'moral division between voluntary and forced mendicancy' (1837: 12).

12 The 'Society against Mendicancy in Rome', founded in 1897 with the aim of helping the 'true' poor and identifying the false ones, was one of the few non-religious organisations dealing with the problem of poverty at the end of the century in Italy.

13 *Discorsi parlamentari del conte Camillo di Cavour, Volume 9*, 1853–1854, p. 142.

14 Speech by Silvio Spaventa to the Italian Chamber of Deputies, 15 June 1880; author's translation from Italian.

15 Ibid.

16 It was not the end of moralisation however. The means-tested pension (applied only to people above 70 years) included a 'behaviour test' aimed at investigating the history of the claimant, including his/her past experiences of idleness and inebriation. This clause was eliminated in 1911 as impracticable.

17 Not incidentally, these policies also included the very first forms of categorical social assistance directed at mothers and children via the introduction of the Protezione della Maternità e dell'Infanzia (National Organisation for the Protection of Motherhood and Infancy). On familialism see Chapter 4 of this book.

18 Mentioned by Mussolini in *Discorso dell'Ascensione*, 26 May 1927.

19 The 'Investigation on destitution and on the means to combat it' was approved by Parliament in 1951 and concluded in 1954.

4 A Trojan Horse?

Public relief at times of crisis

Morality meets austerity

This chapter is centred on the encounter of latent moralising notions of poverty and economic crisis. We will address the case for the 're-moralisation' of the welfare state in recent years (Saunders, 2013). The argument made in the chapter draws upon the idea formulated by Harrison and Sanders (2014) that the set of social policy measures introduced in the UK during recent years operates a sort of 'social control' over the behaviour of welfare claimants. We further expand this notion and anticipate that in many countries welfare programmes are increasingly assuming the traits of a 'Trojan Horse', i.e. a gift given with the tacit intention of accomplishing a hidden plan or agenda. We have learned from anthropological research that gift-giving is always a practice loaded with social norms and cultural meanings (Mauss, 1954; Lévi-Strauss, 1950 [1987]), primarily those regarding assumptions on the obligation to *reciprocate* the giving action. We can agree with Mau (2003) that reciprocity is also a traditional central element of the welfare state, with return expectations on the part of the claimant varying according to each model of social redistribution. However, the increasing introduction of conditionality in the welfare state regulating new expectations in terms of economic and social behaviour of the recipient is transforming the overall social contract of the welfare state. This is particularly evident once we consider that these transformations are eroding the 'social' component of the social contract (i.e. solidarity) and re-enforcing its 'contractual' element. Welfare recipients are increasingly conceived as 'customers' rather than entitled citizens, and social support as a 'temporary' gift that can be withdrawn if social expectations are not met.

So what is the 'hidden' agenda of new welfare programmes? As the above-mentioned study by Harrison and Sanders poignantly illustrates, there is a general attempt at controlling the social behaviour of claimants. However, we can add, the moralisation discourse affecting particular categories of claimants – the undeserving ones – and their assumed 'wrong' behaviour, social and cultural norms is just one more example in the history of poor relief action of a general strategy to discipline the inactive part of the populace and put it to work.

The following sections will be structured as follows: first an analysis of the most recent trends in Britain will be made from the standpoint of the 'Big Society' project and its role as a *moral manifesto* of the Coalition government during the recession. The section will describe how the element of solidarity of public policies addressed at poor and low-income groups has been explicitly excluded from the welfare debate, only to be deceivingly evoked to justify welfare cuts. We will also see how this occurred along with the increasing importance given to individual responsibility as a concept. This will be followed by a description of the Italian context and the emergence of an intergenerational moralising approach toward welfare deservedness.

This section will illustrate how the history of the British welfare state did not necessarily shift 'from individualism to collectivism', as clarified by Lewis (1995: 3), but how it has been characterised by the 'mixed' and different roles of the voluntary sector, the family and the market at different points in time.

The Big Society project: rediscovering solidarity?

On 19 July 2010, at the end of six consecutive quarters of recession, the British Prime Minister, David Cameron, gave what has become one of his most quoted and contested speeches. The topic of this talk was his plan for a 'Big Society', which he described in these terms:

> You can call it liberalism. You can call it empowerment. You can call it freedom. You can call it *responsibility*. I call it the Big Society. The Big Society is about a huge *culture* change [...] where people, in their everyday lives, in their homes, in their neighbourhoods, in their workplace don't always turn to officials, local authorities, or central government for answers to the problems they face, but instead feel both free and powerful enough to *help themselves* and their own communities.[1]

As part of his plan to break with the past government's approach that 'turned *able*, capable individuals into passive recipients of state help with little hope for a better future', the newly elected Coalition leader made the case, among other things, for the devolution of powers to the local levels of government and to an increased engagement of his government to support 'a new *culture* of voluntarism, philanthropy, social action' that could led to the creation of 'neighbourhoods who are in charge of their own destiny'.[2]

For some of his critics, Cameron's enthusiastic call for the construction of a Big Society was 'all about saving money' in a time of austerity, and his plea for a stronger civil society nothing more than a stratagem of the government for 'washing its hands of providing decent public services and using volunteers as a cut-price alternative'.[3] In this regard, the major concern of political opponents, trade unionists, and voluntary and civic organisations alike came precisely from Cameron's emphasis on society's empowerment, the reason being that, notoriously, with *great powers comes great responsibilities*, as also explicitly announced in a policy paper produced by the Cabinet Office.[4] Behind the façade of a new passionate commitment to local communities and civic engagement – and behind the 'we are all in this together' rhetoric – it was contested, Cameron's speech contained, in reality, all the elements for the beginning of a new era of *individualisation* of social risks that could be rather read as 'it's your problem not ours'.[5]

To put it in other words, in the absence of concrete efforts (both financial and political) to implement the Big Society plan, and in conjunction with significant cuts to the public sector, the *wake-up call* on community empowerment risked in fact disrupting social cohesion rather than strengthening it (Davies and Pill, 2012). Political opponents, most notably the Labour Party, were caught off guard by the unprecedented concern of the Conservative wing with societal values and accused them of having 'stolen' their own language of fairness and solidarity to justify cuts at the public sector.[6]

It is only too fitting to look at this narrative as a 'rhetorical device' that created, in the eye of the public, an ideological opposition (the Big Society vs the Big Government) through which the case is made that *more society* and *less state* is the solution for contemporary society's problems (Albrow, 2012: 109). At the same time, it is hard not to analogise Cameron's Big Society project with liberal economist F. A. Hayek's famous views on the advantages of a 'minimal state' (1960) and his critique of the transformation in 'values brought about by the advance of collectivism' responsible for the 'destruction' of typical Anglo-Saxon values such as 'independence and self-reliance, individual initiative and *local responsibility*, the successful reliance on *voluntary activities*' (Hayek, 1944 [2014]: 219, emphasis added).

Cameron's speech on the Big Society is a fundamental point of departure for discussing the encounter of economic crisis and the moralisation of the welfare state during the Great Recession. While officially aimed at reforming the public sector and the overall approach of the so-called 'Big Government's interventions in public life (Corbett and Walker, 2013), the Big Society project is also essentially one of remodelling the state–individual *solidarity* relationships.[7] It is no coincidence, in fact, that the very first public mention of Cameron's Big Society plan, which was made during the election campaign in 2009, was dominated by references to the poverty and welfare debates. Also, and more importantly to our discussion, that speech was profoundly inspired by the belief that by 'undermining personal and social responsibility' 'the big government approach ended up perpetuating poverty instead of solving it',[8] something which echoes back to the Malthusian moralising explanation for the rise of pauperism in the nineteenth century and to the case he made for the abolition of the poor relief.

As Cameron himself declared, it was a *cultural* transformation he hoped for, one that could restore a 'culture of responsibility' and 'activation' among people in their *expectations* in terms of social support from the state, so that the new system can be one that matches 'effort with reward instead of a system that rewards those who make no effort'.[9]

While Cameron warned that the creation of the Big Society culture should not be understood in terms of a 'reheated version of ideological laissez-faire',[10] the new model of solidarity that he outlined has been frequently seen as the necessary precondition – if not justification – for the introduction of a neoliberal agenda (Jacobs and Manzi, 2013). In terms of its approach to social inclusion objectives, it has been noted, the Big Society project came together with the restoration of a 'behaviourist' strategy in social policy (Harrison and Hemingway, 2014) especially directed at the 'broken part' of the British populace:[11] first and foremost, the undeserving poor for whom the new empowering opportunities from the Big Society came hand in hand with the introduction of a 'disciplinary' model of social inclusion.

Recent literature has convincingly demonstrated how the Big Society rhetoric is perfectly consistent with the concrete approach towards social policy over the year of the Great Recession, and in particular with the emergence of new punitive and 'intrusive' (Sanders, 2014: 210) attitude informing welfare reforms addressed to those considered 'undeserving' claimants (Harrison and Sanders, 2014). Examples of such a 'moralising' approach apply to different compartments of the redistribution sphere that have been touched somehow by a new general emphasis on the *give back to society* logic, a welfare ethic regulated by the contractual-based principle that *something must be given in exchange for social benefits*. One of the flagship programmes of this sort is the Mandatory Work Activity Programme. Introduced in June 2011 with a declared intent of enabling individuals to develop 'the discipline and habits of working life',[12] the programme was designed as a compulsory work placement scheme for a 'small number of Jobseeker's Allowance customers who have little or no understanding of what behaviours are required to obtain and keep work' and to help them 'discover for themselves the expectations of work'.[13]

The programme practically introduced the obligation for some jobseekers to earn their benefit by working for free as well, as a new form of conditionality for workers who do not comply with *work ethic* expectations (Berry, 2016).[14] The scheme was greatly criticised for being part of an overall system of sanctions for jobseekers which constrains people to accept unpaid work or to remain 'stuck' in 'low-quality jobs' (Shildrick et al., 2012: 220). More importantly, this and other policy measures introduced during the years of the Great Recession also exemplify the increasing preoccupation of policy-makers with the behaviour of able-bodied claimants: the restoration of the *less-eligibility rule* enforced via the new 'benefit cap' and the recent plan for the introduction of community work for NEETs[15] with the declared purpose of providing them with 'order and discipline'[16] have been widely described as two elements of a 'behavioural' agenda that intends to break welfare 'dependency' by inculcating the 'habit' of work into citizens (Patrick, 2014: 59).

Surely, *contractual* workfare schemes had been introduced by the Labour Party and Tony Blair's New Deal far before the inception of the Great Recession (see Powell, 2008). We can agree in this regard with a large part of the scholarship that the most recent transformations should read as an exacerbation of a long-established trend to combat inactivity by re-enforcing conditionality and individual responsibility (Deacon and Patrick, 2011; MacLeavy, 2011; Harrison and Sanders, 2014). However, it is worth noting that the most recent transformations are distinctive in their strong reliance upon a *moralising discourse* centred on the classification of welfare claimants into different categories and in the symbolic and concrete punishment of those considered 'undeserving' (Lister and Bennett, 2010; Patrick and Brown, 2012; Fletcher, 2015). Part of this trend applies to the latest reforms concerning new rounds of Work Capability Assessment (WCA) performed on disabled recipients and long-term sick persons to test whether they are unfit for work or should be expected to perform working activities, something which has been proved to enforce a logic of suspicion towards this category of claimants and to produce frequent episodes of stigma and marginalisation among the assessed (Garthwaite, 2014; Moffatt and Noble, 2015; Manji, 2016). The extension of this suspicion to categories once considered 'morally untouchable' for their recognised vulnerability – such as the disabled, but also children, asylum seekers and refugees (as noted by Wallace, 2014: 84) – is indicative for many commentators of a qualitative change in the welfare state.

In this regard, it is thus unsurprising to find out that Cameron's appeal to a cultural transformation was also presented as a call for the resolution of a 'moral crisis' (Manzi, 2015). Cameron himself made a very outspoken reference to morality as a fundamental aspect of public policy when he lamented the 'long erosion of responsibility, of social virtue, of self-discipline' and of politicians' general inclination to display a '*moral neutrality*, a refusal to make *judgments* about what is good and bad *behaviour*, right and wrong behaviour', with the risk that no one admits that 'social problems' (among which he mentions poverty, social exclusion, obesity, alcohol abuse, drug addiction) 'are often the consequence of the *choices* that people make'.[17] The emphasis put by David Cameron on the link between individual choices and social problems – and at the same time his insistence on the need of governments and public opinion alike to express their ethical assessment about these themes – ostensibly characterises the Big Society speech as the *moral manifesto* of the Coalition government. Also, they signal the resurgence of a *moralisation of the poor* argument (albeit not always an explicit one) in the political narrative. Some commentators have put into perspective the moralisation dimension of the Big Society narrative and contended that what the project really offered to the public was, in reality, an ideological and psychological strategy to address societal anxieties at a time of profound insecurity (Jacobs, 2015).

Even reformulated in these terms, however, it remains uncertain whether the emphasis put on the spirit of altruism and on 'lost notions of care, mutualism and morality' (Williams et al., 2014: 2800) should be looked at as an invitation to rediscover a (quite romanticised) communitarian past, with the fundamental role of intermediate institutions of solidarity (such as family and local neighbourhood) at the centre of the redistribution model; or, alternatively, as an implicit act of de-responsibilisation of the state to its citizens in the face of increasing social and economic uncertainty. Data from the Office for National Statistics (ONS) on the dramatic increase during the years of the Great Recession of young people aged 20–34 years who live with their parents are suggestive of an unprecedented reliance of the British populace upon family support as a safety net at times of economic crisis.[18]

This is also indicative of the increasing reliance upon informal solidarity. A recent report has indicated, as the first target of a strategy to contrast hunger and 'feed' in Britain, the institution of a network 'composed of the food bank movement and other providers of food assistance' and has praised the work of voluntary organisations committed to this struggle by noting that 'if the Prime Minister wants to meet his Big Society it is here'.[19]

The idea can be perhaps advanced at this point that one of the Big Society's unexpressed objectives is precisely that of returning to the situation of late Victorian times when, notably, poor relief actions were performed more via informal channels of solidarity than through the Poor Law's intervention (Fraser, 1976: 11). As discussed in Chapter 3, at those times, the whole relationship between the governmental level of poor relief (i.e. the Poor Laws system) and philanthropic work constituted a 'microcosm':

> [a] *little-governed* society based essentially on small, local inward looking communities, in which it was very natural for the relief of poverty, like other communal activities, to be primarily organised as *local measures to local problems.*
>
> (McCord, 1976: 109, emphasis added)

It is undeniable that this passage, written far before David Cameron's speech, strikingly resonates with the declared objectives of the 'new' Big Society and puts these two apparently distant worlds in a direct continuity line. This is of major importance for our discussion if we accept the view of most studies, including McCord's quoted above, that the Victorian philanthropic and voluntary world of charity was part and parcel of the Poor Law system. It can be argued that these institutions played a fundamental role not only in complementing the (scarce) institutional actions of relief but also, and more importantly, in transforming the social and moral backgrounds of the British system of solidarity to the needy. Incidentally, these results can be confronted by Mau's 'moral taxonomy' of redistribution systems, with strong conditionality, obligation for reciprocity and prioritisation of self-help corresponding to residual welfare regimes, whose main historical representation remains that the Poor Laws system (2003: 38–40). Finally, at a macroscopic level, the overall Big Society project and the restructuring of solidarity relationships made by the Coalition government can be seen as a Trojan Horse itself that provided citizens with a new set of policy measures to support poverty and joblessness while, at the same time, asking them to resort to informal solidarity, local community and voluntarism for solving their immediate problems.

Generational scroungers in Italy: the *bamboccione* and familism in the Italian context

> We must send those we call *bamboccioni* ('big babies') out of the house.
>
> Tommaso Padoa-Schioppa, October 2007

> Youngsters can't afford to be too choosy [in the labour market] and wait for the 'ideal' job to come.
>
> Elsa Fornero, October 2012

Family has been at the centre of analyses of the Italian model of solidarity for decades now. 'Familialism' (as opposed to familism) – the attribution of a 'maximum of welfare obligations to the household' (Esping-Andersen, 1999: 45) – is said to be one of the most distinctive traits of the Southern European model of social protection (Kohli and Albertini, 2008). In this system, social reliance upon the family as an intermediate actor of social protection is not complemented by public actions encouraging familial care work and its reconciliation with labour activities. Quite the contrary in fact: familialistic welfare systems are characterised by a 'paradoxical' passivity and under-development of family policy (Esping-Andersen, 1999: 51). The Italian variant of this model, which sociologist Chiara Saraceno (2010: 33–34) terms 'unsupported' familialism or 'familialism by default', is historically characterised by high levels of family obligations to the elderly and child care, 'implicitly' supported by generous governmental cash transfer measures for elderly people (Saraceno and Keck, 2010: 692; Ascoli and Pavolini, 2015). For others, the Italian familialism is, in reality, 'explicit' for governmental interventions – or, better, the lack thereof – are intentionally designed to 'strengthen social responsibility among family members' (Leitner, 2003: 356). Regardless of labels, the 'ambivalence' of the Italian model of unsupported familialism, Saraceno points out, can be best explained by looking at the persistence of long-lasting 'cultural' assumptions about family, gender and 'intergenerational responsibilities'. These beliefs do not concern the role of women alone, although they are 'expected to act as a resource of the welfare state'; they also affect the whole idea of family, generally seen as 'social and moral institution' with specific duties in terms of redistribution and social care (Saraceno, 1994: 60, 68).

These accounts of familialism in the Italian model of social protection have revealed the role of the family as a fundamental informal actor of redistribution and solidarity, if not a proper strategic solution against poverty. However, they had also the merit of having put into a different perspective the role of kin relationships as depicted by Edward C. Banfield's 'amoral familism'. In researching the origins of 'backwardness' and poverty in a small southern Italian rural village he names 'Montegrano',[20] Banfield famously advanced his 'predictive hypothesis' that the condition of the Montegranesi could be predominantly attributed to their *ethos* and abnormal 'state of *culture*' centred on their kin relationship that prevents them from furthering group and community interests and for contributing to the public good (Banfield, 1958: 155, emphasis added). As a result of their 'cultural lag', Banfield posits, these people are 'prisoners of their family-centred ethos, [...] a fundamental impediment to their economic and other progress' so embedded within them that it could be 'perpetuated' for a long time despite changing circumstances (ibid.: 160).[21]

Banfield's work has been subject to much scrutiny and criticism over the years (Silverman, 1968; Miller, 1974; Muraskin, 1974). Most contemporary studies now agree that it contributed to the production of 'a false paradigm' (Ferragina, 2009: 142): that the specific nature of family relationships in rural Italian communities could be read as a condition that delayed their economic and social development (Leonardi, 1995). Also, Banfield's work diffused the (distorted) idea that kin sense of solidarity among southern Italians is 'amoral', as intrinsically opposed to a morality of community good. Banfield most likely conceived the whole Montegrano poor community as 'undeserving' of social support, as primarily responsible for its own misfortune – or, as he would put it, for their misery. Yet, as distorted as this may have been, Banfield's interpretation of poverty and its origins in the Italian context can be instrumental to the analysis of the Italian model of social support. On the one hand, Banfield's work is at least indicative of the belated acknowledgement, in Italy as elsewhere in the world, of scientific explanations of poverty and its causes. At the same time however, it tells us much in terms of the *misinterpreted* role of family and kin relationships as one of the most important channels of solidarity and redistribution in Italy.

A classic theme that is generally debated when family relationships and social safety net are taken into account is that of the Italian *bamboccione*. This section opened with two quotes made by previous members of the Italian government, respectively former Economics Minister Tommaso Padoa-Schioppa and former Welfare Minister Elsa Fornero. Reference is made in these quotes to the figure of the *bamboccione* – literally 'big babies' – and to their placement in the labour market in terms of a 'cultural' problem, the assumption being that it is predominantly Italian young adults who choose to live with their parents and stay unemployed. As mentioned above, in Italy there is a strong tradition of familial networks of social support, a channel of redistribution and social protection which frequently complements – not to say substitutes – social policy measures or services. Among the diverse forms of social support made by parents, grandparents, children and extended families, a significant role has been traditionally played by cohabitation patterns in Italian families.[22] The proportion of young adults living with parents has always been very high in Italy, something that can be attributed to a number of causes: the persistence of social and religious norms; the diffusion of high levels of educational attainment which in turn delay entrance into the labour market; but also, and predominantly, economic and labour market insecurity for an increasingly greater part of young adults. Research conducted in 2009 reveals that 41.9 per cent of people between 18 and 34 years living with parents attribute the cause of their situation to economic difficulties (Istat, 2014). If living with parents can be considered a form of survival strategy for young people trying to 'get on their feet' in the labour market before moving out of the nest, it goes without saying that the inception of the Great Recession in Italy has only added to the need for many families to adopt coping strategies that involve cohabitation and family support, as the comparison displayed in Figures 4.1 and 4.2 below illustrates.

However, it is interesting to note that the whole moralisation discourse made in the previous section of this chapter with reference to the British case can be applied, in the Italian context, to the generational model of redistribution and solidarity. Declarations such as those made by Elsa Fornero

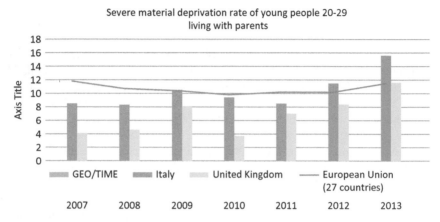

Figure 4.1 Severe material deprivation rates for young people aged 20–29 and living with parents, 2007–2013
Source: Author's calculation from Eurostat data, 2015.

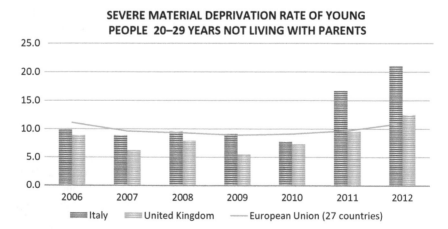

Figure 4.2 Severe material deprivation rates for young people aged 20–29 years not living with parents, 2007–2013
Source: Author's calculation from Eurostat data, 2015.

and Tommaso Padoa-Schioppa are quintessential of a new general inclination to point at young adults as 'choosy', lazy or just 'mama's boys', a rhetoric that has assumed a strong 'moralising' tone especially during the years of the economic crisis (see Censis, 2012). It is in fact not incidental that these two declarations, which attracted mounting protest among the public, emerged in conjunction with the introduction of severe austerity measures in the Italian welfare state. As for the British case, this narrative can be understood in terms of an overall critique of an assumed 'culture' of laziness ascribed to young Italian adults that must be contrasted by encouraging them to enter the labour market at a time of economic crisis.

If one wanted to apply the general deservedness discourse to this topic, we could say that the Italian *bamboccione* are increasingly represented as the quintessence of the 'voluntary unemployed' who sponge off society of its resources. This, however, occurs in spite of the evident lack of welfare resources addressed to young people in Italy and in the face of living condition figures such those presented above. At the same time, the Trojan Horse argument made for the British case can be also applied to the Italian context. Welfare reforms introduced during the years of the crisis in Italy seem to be informed by a reconfiguration of the social contract which is not too different from the one we found in Britain. As elsewhere in Europe and in the world, social assistance plans make now explicit reference to a list of expected behaviours on the part of the claimant. In order to be eligible to receive the *carta acquisti* (€400 per month),[23] recipients are obliged to sign an agreement requesting that family members: establish regular contact with the local welfare office; engage in the active search for a job; participate in training and job placement; ensure school attendance for children; and commit to healthcare and prevention activities.

Metaphors and self-fulfilling prophecies

We conclude this chapter by looking at the topics examined here in a comparative perspective. Certainly, the British and Italian cases are perhaps too different to allow us to perform such a comparison in a systematic fashion, especially in their very different social and economic backgrounds but most importantly in the diverse extent of the public and political discussion which is made in these two countries around the 'function' of welfare state and solidarity. However, if a conclusion can be drawn from the discussion made in this chapter, it certainly concerns the role of solidarity. Regardless of the historical models of redistribution and public relief existing in the two countries, it can be said that the recent global crisis did create room for the rise of a certain 'moral panic' around the welfare systems in place. In both Britain and Italy, the emergence of austerity requirements has urged the need to rethink priorities and to 'rebalance' the distribution of resources among the different segments of society first and foremost according to normative schemes (Hemerijck, 2013). This 'brainstorming' operation in the public sphere has resulted in the re-enforcement (or reconfiguration) of boundaries between deserving and undeserving categories of claimants. In some cases, it even took the form of a (partial) disruption of the post-war social contract made between the state and its citizens, with the solidarity element of institutional redistribution giving way to its contractual component.

The provocative metaphor of welfare benefits as a Trojan Horse is probably unfair to the fundamental role that social policy still plays in many European countries, but it can be seen as a fitting interpretation of the exacerbation of the contractual dimension in the welfare state. At the same it is possible to look at the two different patterns observed in this chapter from the perspective of their effects. Surprisingly, and despite their profound historical differences, in the aftermath of the Great Recession the Italian and the British cases seem to realise a 'self-fulfilling prophecy' (Merton, 1948). The case made two years into the global crisis for a new role to be played by the so-called Big Society in Britain has resulted in an increased and 'forced' reliance of families and individuals upon kinship relationships and informal channels of support, such as food banks, charities and voluntary organisations. At the same time, the Italian case shows that the continuing lack of political commitment towards the establishment of public poor relief actions – coupled with certain cultural assumptions concerning young people, the family and its responsibilities – has only amplified the perpetuation of a distinctive form of 'forced familism' in times of crisis (Gambardella and Morlicchio, 2005).

Notes

1 Official transcript of the speech given by PM David Cameron at Liverpool Hope University, 19 July 2010 (emphasis added). Full text available at www.gov.uk/government/speeches/big-society-speech.
2 Ibid.
3 Declaration of General Secretary of the trade union UNISON, Dave Prentis, BBC, 19 July 2010.
4 'Building the Big Society', published by the Cabinet Office, 18 May 2010, available at www.gov.uk/government/publications/building-the-big-society.
5 Extract from the speech of Tessa Jowell, Shadow Minister for the Olympics, to the 2010 Labour Party conference, available at www2.labour.org.uk/tessa-jowells-speech-to-labour-party-conference.
6 A number of commentators contrasted Margaret Thatcher's famous quote – that 'there is no such thing as society' (and David Cameron's own almost identical declaration in 2008) – with the new emphasis on the Big Society as an incoherent deviation from the Conservatives' political identity (Dorey, 2015). In reality, on that very occasion Margaret Thatcher also made the following comment, which is striking for its similarity to the ideas expressed by Cameron in 2010: 'Too many people have been given to understand that if they have a problem, it's the government's job to cope with it. "I have a problem, I'll get a grant." "I'm homeless, the government must house me"' (interview with *Women's Own* magazine, 31 October 1987).
7 For an in-depth discussion on the role of libertarian paternalism as one of the political and philosophical roots of the Big Society project see Corbett and Walker, 2013.

8 Extract from David Cameron's Hugo Young lecture, given at Kings Place in London, 9 November 2009. Full text available at http://conservative-speeches.sayit. mysociety.org/speech/601246.

9 David Cameron's speech, 23 May 2011. Full text available at www.gov.uk/government/ speeches/speech-on-the-big-society.

10 Hugo Young lecture, 2009.

11 David Cameron speech, 14 February 2011. Full text available at www.gov.uk/ government/speeches/pms-speech-on-big-society.

12 Mandatory Work Activity Provider Guidance: Incorporating Universal Credit (UC) Guidance (April 2014), available at www.gov.uk/government/uploads/system/ uploads/attachment_data/file/300734/pg-part-p.pdf.

13 Department for Work and Pensions, Mandatory Work Activity: Equality Impact Assessment (March 2011), available at www.gov.uk/government/uploads/system/ uploads/attachment_data/file/220276/eia-mandatory-work-activity.pdf.

14 Jobseekers failing to participate in or complete the programme undergo sanctions (suspension of the benefit for 13 weeks). A second failure during the next 12 months results in a 26-week sanction.

15 Young people not in education, employment or training.

16 Declaration of Prime Minister David Cameron, quoted on the BBC, 17 February 2015.

17 David Cameron speech at Glasgow, 7 July 2008, emphasis added. Full text available at www.telegraph.co.uk/news/politics/conservative/2263705/David-Cameron-attacks-UK-moral-neutrality-full-text.html.

18 Data published in 2014, available at http://webarchive.nationalarchives.gov.uk/ 20160105160709; www.ons.gov.uk/ons/rel/family-demography/young-adults-living-with-parents/2013/sty-young-adults.html.

19 'Feeding Britain: a strategy for zero hunger in England, Wales, Scotland and Northern Ireland', All-Party Parliamentary Inquiry into Hunger in the United Kingdom (2014: 17), available at https://feedingbritain.files.wordpress.com/2015/02/ food-poverty-feeding-britain-final-2.pdf.

20 This is the fictional name he uses for Chiaromonte, a village in the Basilicata region. Significantly, Banfield makes abundant use of the Italian word *miseria* in his text, as if to stress that the condition of material destitution among the inhabitants of Montegrano is also accompanied by a status of squalor and 'chronic melancholy' that Banfield attributes to their 'culture' and to 'social and biological deprivations' (1958: 63, 65).

21 Among the prospective methods that could successfully change the ethos of Montegranesi, Banfield proposed the introduction of Protestantism, which in other cases (he mentions Brazil) proved capable of reducing 'illiteracy, dishonesty and gambling' (1958: 162). Elsewhere in the text Banfield read Montegrano's ethos and lack of organization through Weber's interpretation of Protestantism as a major force in the development of capitalism (ibid.: 87).

22 For a discussion of the Italian case in a comparative perspective see Paci and Pugliese (2011) or Ascoli and Pavolini (2015).

23 We refer to the last round of experimentation of the social card, which was introduced in 2013 and which is expected to be substituted by a new card in 2017.

Part II
Narratives of deservedness

5   Under the limelight

'Parasites', 'scroungers' and 'welfare queens'

From moral to socio-economic deviance: the popularisation of deservedness

In his famous volume on the 'undeserving poor' in America, Michael B. Katz (1990 [2013]: 1) identifies three great questions that mark any debate on poverty: how to 'draw boundaries' between deserving and undeserving claimants; how to avoid the 'dependence' of those receiving support; what are the 'limits' of solidarity and collective responsibility. Discussions on these themes, as we saw in the last two chapters, have been for some time almost the exclusive pre-rogative of dominant groups (governments, intellectuals, reformers) whose visions, in fact, shaped and informed collective ideas and representations of poverty and social responsibility towards the poor. It is true, as previous chapters have documented, that the notion of the undeserving poor is a recurrent and almost universal theme in the history of humanity. However, what chiefly characterises its contemporary version is the 'public' dimension that it has assumed over the last century. The three problems identified by Katz today are a matter of discussion and interest not only for governments and intellectuals but also, and increasingly so, for the general public. Factors such as universal suffrage, the emergence of social security schemes that transformed the majority of the population into contributors to the welfare system, mass education, trade unionism, economic and political lobbying and the increasing influence of the media have pushed the issue of the undeserving poor into the limelight.

The history of relief and solidarity towards the needy, as the first part of this book illustrated, reveals the convenient and recurrent use made by govern-ments of negative *social categorisations* of the undeserving poor for political, economic and social purposes. Is this still the case? The answer of course, is yes. But we must also remember that this process is no longer unidirectional. Public opinion – i.e. *voters* – does shape to a large extent governments' political agendas today, and especially so in the domain of welfare programmes, social justice and redistribution. Public opinion and its preference for expanding, rather than diminishing, public spending trajectories, for example, has been widely considered to be one of the main explanations for the resistance of the welfare state to profound transformations in the direction of retrenchment, even in the face of significant economic constraints (Pierson, 1994; Pierson, 1996; Brooks and Manza, 2006).[1]

Having clarified the bidirectional relationships regulating public opinion and government welfare agendas, we can now look at the important question of how public opinion on deservedness and solidarity is informed not only by governments' *actions* but also by political narratives and media representations.

Most scholars acquainted with the sociology of knowledge recognise that reality is 'a social construction' (Berger and Luckmann, 1967) built upon cultural representations that shape our perceptions and reinforce our beliefs concerning a certain issue. Cultural studies have long discussed how the media contribute to the construction of a given social reality (Hall, 1980; Gamson et al., 1992) and have evidenced their salient role in the social representation of ideologies, norms and values produced by dominant groups. Likewise, most scholars have come to agree that poverty is not a neutral phenomenon and that it is always socially constructed upon values, culture(s) and cultural representations (Schneider and Ingram, 2005; O'Connor, 2002; van Oorschot et al., 2008).

If poverty can be said to be a social product, there is sufficient evidence to affirm that it is also significantly constituted by *social representations*, understood as 'means of constructing reality' that create 'the substratum of common sense' and give shape to myths (Moscovici, 1988: 216, 230). Far from being abstract objects, negative stereotyped categorisations of the welfare claimant population in terms of being 'undeserving' materialise in a number of ways: they bring about detrimental psychological effects on individuals in terms of shame (Lister, 2004) that add up to the stigmatising dimension of certain social-assistance practices (Pellissery et al., 2014); they can exacerbate societal divisions and feed and re-enforce public misconceptions. It is therefore of major importance for the present discussion to understand how political rhetoric and media narratives have produced and reinforced certain social representations of the undeserving poor in contemporary society.

This chapter will address the theme of social representations of the undeserving poor by looking at three 'mythological' personifications of this category in the public sphere. The 'parasite', the 'scrounger' and the 'welfare queen' emerged in three different contexts: in pre-1989 socialist countries, in 1970s' Britain and the US in the 1980s respectively. Interestingly, these social categories are the specific products not only of political rhetoric and propaganda but also of stereotyped representations produced by the media. In this perspective, the parasite, the scrounger and the welfare queen can be understood as 'modern evolutions' of the past archetype of undeserving poor, the idle pauper. The cases discussed below are indicative of two peculiar but characteristic traits of contemporary narratives about solidarity and deservedness: the transition from a public rhetoric centred on the assumed 'immoral' deviation of the undeserving poor to their characterisation in terms of a social and economic 'burden' on society as a whole.

The *burden argument* is by no means new. However, what is distinctive is the *popularisation* of such an argument and the increasing level of public concern for cases of abuse of the welfare system. This phase began during the second half of the nineteenth century, a period during which old representations of the undeserving poor based on cultural and moral shortcomings began to be replaced by descriptions made in terms of 'parasites', 'spongers' or 'scroungers': resentment of those suspected of depriving society of *economic resources* began to replace the past fear of the undeserving poor as a 'moral and sanitary' menace to the collective. Increasingly over the last decades, the main characteristics of these two arguments is their emergence in times of 'moral panic' and economic crisis, and the recurrent branding of the undeserving poor as criminal, immoral and lazy. The eruption of the 'scroungerphobia' case of Britain in the 1970s, which will be discussed below, is a good example of this trend.

The socialist 'parasite'

By the beginning of the Second World War, as mentioned in Chapter 3, the old notion that poverty was essentially a result of individual behaviour and strongly associated with idleness and crime began to be broadly questioned in most parts of Europe. The appearance of the first studies on unemployment, underemployment and casual labour, among other things, paved the way for a gradual recognition of the complex and multifaceted relationships existing between poverty and labour market exclusion (Jahoda et al., 1971). At the same time, the economic and social development of most European countries, coupled with the expansion of social security systems, significantly reduced the scope of the debate on poverty in Europe, boosting the belief that the giant of 'Want' had been eliminated (Townsend, 1962). While this process occurred in most Western European nations, this was not the case beyond the Iron Curtain. In communist countries the *illusion* (Woodward, 1995) of full employment became the 'established norm' (Moskoff, 1992) and made poverty and unemployment politically inconceivable. In most of the countries under communist rule, not only would public discussion of poverty generally be banned (Wiles and Markowski, 1971; Szelenyi, 1983; Dziewiecka-Bokun, 2000) but also the very existence of poverty itself was denied, and certain kinds of welfare programmes (most notably unemployment and social assistance schemes) were accordingly eliminated since they were deemed *unnecessary*.

As part of its attempt to affirm such an ideological illusion, communist propaganda promulgated the idea of unemployment as a 'parasite' activity, inherently linked to idleness and political dissidence. The identification of the able-bodied individual as undeserving of support and potentially 'dangerous' for society became a common theme in most countries of the communist bloc, where the social rule existed that 'he who does not work shall not eat'. This was especially evident in Soviet countries, where itinerants, 'gypsies', beggars, orphans and those who 'refused' to participate in socially useful work were publicly described as 'parasitical' and 'socially dangerous elements' (Fitzpatrick, 2006: 379). In most Soviet countries the able-bodied unemployed person was not simply a particular category of undeserving poor: labour inactivity was described as an 'explicit anti-social choice' (Milanovic, 1995: 4–5) and even subject to persecution by the authorities at least from the 1930s onwards, when the penalisation of idleness was first introduced. Hostility to and persecution of voluntary unemployment in the communist bloc have been widely understood not so much as a reaction to a specific case of economic crisis, but rather as part and parcel of the ongoing communist attempt at overcoming the deficiencies of the planned economy, above all the *shortage* of labour in certain regions of the USSR (Kornai, 1992).

Needless to say, although it was essentially an economic strategy – explicitly admitted by the governments themselves (as noted by Callum, 1995) – communist anti-parasitism was full of references to the assumed 'immoral' and 'asocial' character of these deviants. Moreover, the negative moralising narrative regarding the parasites was not only found in political speeches. Soviet propaganda made consistent use of visual tools, most notably posters, to glorify the worker icon as part of a mass campaign in support of pro-ductivity (Bonnell, 1997: 36). The rhetoric in favour of the worker *hero* was predictably complemented by visual campaigns against its greatest antithesis: the unemployed. Unsurprisingly, Soviet posters frequently condemned inactive individuals as parasites who refused to work or as frauds intentionally cheating the system. One piece of artwork from 1931, for example, portrays the typical Hercules-like worker. The poster's caption, which reads 'Parasites and slackers do nothing and prevent others from working', is indicative of an important aspect of the treatment of parasites under communism: the *incitement to public hostility* against them and the constant attempt to involve the popula-tion in the accusation and condemnation of persons suspected of living parasitically. This process, which Callum (1995: 14) terms 'the popularisation' of parasites' legal punishment, found its culmination in conjunction with the USSR's Anti-Parasite Laws of the late 1950s which regulated the public *ostracism* of parasite neighbours, officially decided via the 'social sentence' of people's assemblies.[2]

This phenomenon grew further during the 1960s when new laws legitimised the punishment (i.e. deportation) of those accused of being unemployed.[3] In 1983, just a few years before the fall of the Iron Curtain, some 90,000 people were prosecuted as 'parasites' (Granick, 1987). Reportedly, the 'social' com-ponent of the parasites' penalisation came to be abused by landowners and local communities, who tended 'to expel not only the immoral and insolent but also the aged and infirm' (Beermann, 1964: 421). In fact, quite unusually in the history of the undeserving poor, the Soviet attack on this category was exceptionally extended to the *disabled*. They were frequently depicted in posters and movies as dependent parasites, frauds and even accused of being responsible for their own condition (Iarskaia-Smirnova and Romanov, 2014). We have mentioned already that one of the social 'functions' of the undeserving poor in almost all societies is that of providing a constant reminder about the limits of permissible behaviour.

While the case of the social penalisation of idleness under communist rule is only presented here for the purpose of description, it is a fitting example of three characteristics of the undeserving poor: firstly, the 'deliberate marginalisation' of socially deviant individuals (Zubkova, 2010: 14), including those accused of being parasites, was a *social reminder* of what forms of behaviour were not accepted within the communist system (in this particular case, labour inactivity and vagrancy), thus acting to reinforce the established norm in terms of solidarity and support ('He who does not work shall not eat') for the whole population. Secondly, it provided both the public and the communist governments with a *convenient scapegoat* for the economic and political shortcomings of the system. Thirdly, the myth of the communist parasite perfectly exemplifies how dominant groups may actively contribute to construct a social reality (the unemployed understood as being deviant and dangerous elements of society) by means of what Althusser (2006: 92) would refer to as 'Ideological State Apparatuses' (soviet propaganda).

The British 'scrounger'

Is it true that the issue of the undeserving poor faded from public discourse during the *Trente Glorieuses* of the welfare state? Probably yes, at least in terms of explicit references to this topic. However, a distinction should be made concerning the treatment of the undeserving claimant in different 'worlds of welfare capitalism' (Esping-Andersen, 1990). It is certainly true, albeit for very different reasons, that in both social democratic countries of Northern Europe and in former communist countries the explicit discussion about deservedness in the welfare state became more peripheral during this period. This was not the case, by contrast, in the 'liberal' world (primarily in the UK and the US), where the end of the *Trente Glorieuses* and the inception of the 'crisis of welfare capitalism' (Mishra, 1984) exacerbated the public concern about cases of 'voluntary unemployment'. This was especially the case in Britain, where a 'scrounger hunt' on the part of social workers was initiated as early as the beginning of the 1970s (Picton, 1975; Seyd, 1976; Whittington, 1977). By the end of the decade, however, the 'anti-scrounger' campaign became a matter of public relevance, with the media adding to the clamour. At that time, the coverage of welfare fraud cases in the British press was so intensive, even 'hysterical' (Golding and Middleton, 1979: 6), that public anxiety over this matter swiftly assumed the aspect of what Alan Deacon has termed a proper 'scroungerphobia' (1978: 122).

However, and more importantly for our discussion, Golding and Middleton (1982: 237) also noted that media coverage only amplified 'latent' social anxieties and 'ideological' preoccupations with the 'scrounger' phenomenon that were already part of the British social system. Not surprisingly, concerns about welfare abuses became even more prevalent after the British media reported the arrest of Derek Peter Deevy, a 41-year-old social security fraudster 'with 41 names [...] a luxury lifestyle', spending '£25 a week on cigars' and who admittedly had obtained 'a total of £36,000 by fraud'.[4] Studies on British scroungerphobia have generally agreed on the pivotal role of certain media in amplifying the anxiety of the public on this and other cases of welfare fraud. Deacon himself wondered whether the growing concern expressed by British public opinion was 'a rational response' to the press coverage of Deevy and similar cases, and suggested that it could rather have been explained as a 'deep-rooted hostility to the unemployed which becomes more intense in periods of recession and is then reflected and further inflamed in the press' (Deacon, 1978: 127).

In a similar vein, the study conducted by Golding and Middleton (1979) on the UK press coverage revealed that in this particular period popular journalism began to devote an exceptional amount of space to unemployment dole fraud cases as compared to welfare news concerning pensions and family benefits. Discussion of single cases of local dole fraudsters, not surprisingly, was accompanied by increasing attention to and public controversy over the 'alarming proportion' of welfare abuses, which sparked a new debate on the required transformation of the overall social security system and its loopholes. Expressions of concern that thousands of Britons have been shown 'to take advantage of the 30-year-old Womb-to-tomb national security system'[5] reportedly exaggerated the real proportions of the phenomenon of fraud and nurtured the belief that the British welfare system had become 'one of the biggest rackets' in the country, 'cheating the honest tax-payer' and 'the truly deserving cases'.[6] While it is true that different newspapers emphasised the need to keep the system in place in order to guarantee assistance to those in need, the bulk of the discussion soon focussed on the need to identify the *honest welfare claimant* and accordingly the old distinction between deserving and undeserving categories of poor was called for. At the same time, the need to reduce work disincentives in the social security system (i.e. decreasing the extent of unemployment benefits) became an urgent issue in the political agenda, marking the revival of the 'less-eligibility' mechanism in the welfare state.

This latter point is of major importance to our discussion, as it sheds light on the relationship between public scroungerphobia, economic crises and the reactions of governments to the welfare abuse debate. Even if most scholars agree that the turning point in British 'welfare retrenchment' only came in the early 1980s (Pierson, 1994; Hicks, 1999), the revival of the scrounger myth and the ensuing debate resulted in (or at least paralleled) the introduction of a much stricter control over welfare eligibility. It is no surprise that the whole scrounger 'hysteria' exploded in 1976, when, following the onset of a deep financial crisis, Britain had to opt for an International Monetary Fund (IMF) loan, which was conditional upon the introduction of public-spending cuts. Needless to say, the welfare abuse alarm propagated by the media eventually paved the way for the call for the severe restructuring of the expensive welfare system. As a result, under the Callaghan government prosecutions for fraud not only increased to 25,000 cases in one year (1977), but also public welfare spending cuts were introduced, paving the way for a new age of welfare austerity.

The 'welfare queen'

If the existence of the undeserving poor can be said to be a fundamental element of the welfare system, the US is probably one of the countries where this mechanism is the most visible, and where both the treatment and the social depiction of the poor are profoundly reflected in moralising categorisations/representations of claimants. One of the recurrent critiques of the US welfare state is that it lies on deserving/undeserving dichotomies that are 'inextricably linked' (Levenstein, 2004: 226) to the symbolic and ethical meanings of two distinctive dimensions: race and gender (Gordon, 1990; Gordon, 2001; Massey, 2007). A typical element of the US approach to poverty, the incorporation of single mothers into the undeserving poor category (Gordon, 1992; de Acosta, 1997) has been described as a 'backlash against feminism' and women's rights, with the US welfare mother becoming an 'undeserving, lazy, dependent, irresponsible, oversexed' figure, rather than a vulnerable potential recipient of social support (Law, 1983; McCormack, 2004: 358). Parallel to this process, as sociologist Jill Quadagno illustrates, the whole construction of social security institutions in the US has also historically encouraged the enforcement of a 'racial welfare state regime' (1994: 19). These accounts, and the vast literature concerning the 'racialisation' and 'feminisation' of poverty and inequality in the North American system, are indicative of the fact that the overall deservedness definition in the US, and the narratives regarding it, are significantly different from those experienced by most European countries.

As was the case in other industrialised countries, in the US the debate on poverty was temporarily dismissed during the post-war economic growth and only 'rediscovered' in the 1960s.[7] Together with this discovery however, as Michael Katz (1990: 14) claims, also came the 'appropriation', by the conservative wing, of the 'culture of poverty' argument made by Oscar Lewis (1959) (see Chapter 2). In such an appropriation, a fundamental role was played by studies inspired by Lewis's argument. Focusing on an alleged relationship between the diffusion of urban 'ghettos' in northern cities of the country and an apparently distinctive subculture of 'negro poverty' (Harrington, 1962: 63), these studies paved the way for the popularisation and politicisation of the 'subculture' argument, which became a fitting 'modern academic label for the undeserving poor' (Katz, 1990: 14) and their alleged socially deviant behaviour.[8]

One peculiar characteristic of the US is the strong interconnection between political narratives, media representations and public attitudes towards the undeserving poor. As a result of the above-mentioned dynamics, from the 1970s on the typical undeserving poor became increasingly more associated with a particular stereotyped category of welfare claimant: the black, single mother, dependent on the welfare state and with an 'uncontrolled sexuality' (Fraser and Gordon, 1994: 311). These representations, as the study by Martin Gilens (1996) shows, were vigorously promoted by the media: TV and weekly magazines, he notes, not only re-enforced popular representations of undeserving poor but also produced a profound discrepancy between the portrayals of the poor and the very nature of poverty in the US. The over-representation of both African-American and the undeserving poor in media coverage of welfare fraud cases eventually found its personalisation in the American *welfare queen* archetype. Stereotypical representations of welfare queens gained currency during the 1970s and the 1980s, popularised by newspapers and magazines – especially after Ronald Reagan had coined the term in 1976, when he denounced the story of a Chicago black woman reportedly arrested for having cheated on the welfare system, described as having:

> 80 names, 30 addresses, 12 Social Security cards […] collecting veterans' benefits on four non-existing deceased husbands. […] She's got Medicaid, getting food stamps and she is collecting welfare under each of her names. Her tax-free cash income alone is over $150,000.[9]

Reagan would repeatedly use this story when debating welfare issues during his mandate (1981–1985). In fact, the welfare queen myth became part and parcel of the whole anti-welfare rhetoric invoked by both Reagan and the conservative US media in their attack on the 'welfare culture', indicated as one major determinant of poverty and unemployment in the country. The welfare queen anecdote played a central role in promoting the belief that people living on benefits would intentionally exploit the system: the specific case of the Chicago woman with her reported fraud accusations emphasised the 'criminal' behaviour of the undeserving poor.

Predictably, the welfare queen story contributed to the perpetuation of the old stereotype of African-Americans as 'poor and lazy' and fuelled the overall opposition of the US population to 'permissive' welfare programmes (Gilens, 1996: 118). The myth of the welfare queen(s) and the public concern for welfare abuses committed by (African-American) social benefit 'impostors' became so embedded in US public opinion that it was still alive by the end of the 1990s, as recent research has shown (Valentino et al., 2002; Hancock, 2004; Rose and Baumgartner, 2013).

As was the case with other undeserving stereotypes discussed in this chapter, the welfare queen myth surfaced in a time of moral panic for US society. It is perhaps no coincidence that the very first reference to the welfare queen story appeared in 1976, in conjunction with a severe financial crisis and, even more importantly, at a time when the expansion of social and civic rights had made welfare expenditure unsustainable. The cost of the principal social welfare scheme (Aid to families with dependent children) rose incredibly, from $4.8 billion in 1970 to $9.2 billion in 1975 (Handler and Hasenfeld, 1991: 113), predominantly (but not exclusively) as an effect of the increased participation of unmarried black women in the programme.[10] Not incidentally, single mothers became the target of increasing attacks in both political and scientific arenas alike. These attacks would point the finger precisely at the existing welfare system for having created a culture of 'dependence' and a 'poverty trap' among those receiving support (Murray, 1984), reinvigorating the old pauperisation argument and the case for the abolition of indiscriminate support to the undeserving poor.

Regardless of the success of Reagan's attempt at 'dismantling' the welfare state (Pierson, 1994) and regardless of whether or not the Chicago woman story was a made-up anecdote used by the New Right to legitimise the war on 'welfare dependence' and its retrenchment actions, the invention of the welfare queen stereotype proved to be significant in political terms. As Michael Katz points out, a major factor in the conservatives' triumph in the 1980s was precisely their 'convincing' criticism of the undeserving poor, which provided the population with an 'explanation for economic stagnation and moral decay' (1990: 167) and legitimised a true 'politics of disgust' enforced against stereotyped undeserving welfare claimants (Hancock, 2004).

The lives of others: the 'spectacularisation' of poverty

Ask someone what the first thing is that comes into their mind when hearing the word 'welfare' and a number of images will immediately arise. Increasingly over the last number of years, those images very often portray common situations: A young man drinking a beer in the street in the middle of the day. A woman complaining about the lack of local job opportunities and lamenting her inability to pay the rent while holding two different brand-new iPhones in her hands. A (possibly) recovering drug addict withdrawing his weekly benefit payment from an ATM, only to contact the local drug dealer a few minutes later to arrange a meeting. A recently arrived Roma family from Romania collecting scrap metal from the bins, leaving the whole street littered with garbage. A welfare fraudster who fiddles his benefits by just going about his daily job – shoplifting.

Not incidentally, these images resonate with those portrayed on the first episode of *Benefits Street*, a documentary/reality show broadcast by the British Channel 4. The programme describes the lives of residents of James Turner Street in Birmingham. Here the majority of the inhabitants are reportedly unemployed and live off welfare benefits. The show was first broadcast in early January 2014, proving to be highly successful and immediately provoking heated controversy.[11] Local residents protested against the show's negative representation of their neighbourhood and demanded the programme's immediate removal. Several (especially, but not exclusively, left-wing) commentators at the same time severely criticised the stigmatising effects of the show on the representation of the welfare recipient population, pointing out that the description of James Turner Street's residents provided by Channel 4 intentionally emphasises and encourages the stereotype of the welfare 'parasite', undeservingly living off and wasting welfare benefits on drugs, alcohol and luxury items, as well as the assumed inclination to crime and poor lifestyle choices.

The broadcast of *Benefits Street* is indicative of a wider phenomenon (in the UK and other countries): the diffusion, during recent years, of factual TV shows centred on the lifestyles and attitudes of welfare recipients, thus popularizing themes such as poverty, benefit fraud, dependency and deservedness in the welfare system. The obsession of the media with the lives of the poor has come to the point that a series titled *Famous, Rich and Hungry* (BBC, 2014) came out, documenting the experience of 'four famous volunteers' who lived for three days with 'families who can't afford to eat'.[12] *Guardian* journalist Barbara Ellen poignantly summarised the whole intent of the programme as a 'safari experience' at the end of which the stars featured in the show (including Rachel Johnson, journalist and younger sister of former London mayor Boris Johnson) would go 'home to feel relieved that they weren't poor', leaving their hosts remaining poor – 'just a little more televised'.[13]

A central point in the debate over the role of *Benefits Street* and likeminded TV programmes, Ellen's final remark is central to our discussion. The *spectacularisation* of poverty and people living in poverty (and of those whose survival depends on welfare support) is strictly linked to the moral dimension of poverty and solidarity at different levels. Firstly, it is a major component of the process mentioned at the beginning of this chapter, which is the gradual transformation of 'deservedness' into an issue of interest for the general public and whose most recent manifestation is precisely that the undeserving poor have once more come under media scrutiny. The broadcast of programmes like those mentioned above elicits opinions and discussion among the general public on who should be considered 'deserving' in a given society. As such, these TV shows might be said to have a double effect: on the one hand, they disclose the extent to which welfare cuts have exposed people to poverty and marginalisation, especially during the years of the Great Recession. At the same time however, and increasingly so, the stereotyped and oversimplified representation of welfare claimants and their lifestyles has unleashed attacks on different categories of welfare recipients and has legitimised a narrative that 'frames' the poor and identifies the undeserving claimant as the most immediate scapegoat to blame during the crisis (Garland, 2014; Beresford, 2016).

At the same time, however, the popularisation of poverty and welfare deservedness as public issues is but one element of a much wider process characteristic of post-modernity – the appropriation and consequent spectacularisation of 'suffering' experiences (Kleinman and Kleinman, 1996: 1–2) that are 'used as a commodity' to 'appeal emotionally and morally' to the audience and that have become subject to a 'cultural representation' through which the suffering experience itself is 'remade, thinned out, and distorted'. When we consider media representations of *poverty* in particular, however, a question needs to be asked. Unlike journalistic coverage of sensational human experiences of suffering – such as those provoked by war, famine, epidemics or ecological disasters – the spectacularisation of poverty such as in *Benefits Street* relies on 'ordinary' and intimate life stories. On the one hand, it might indeed be claimed that these programmes do not even *document* poverty, as they rather fall within the category of 'fiction'; thus their spectacularisation could not be justified as an instrument of public information. However, other commentators note, it would be a mistake to consider *Benefits Street* and like-minded TV products as purely fiction, the lives of those portrayed being real and subject to real suffering. Watching these programmes as though they were fictional products according to the critics is essentially immoral: you just cannot sit and wait for season number two.

Whether fiction or not, most critics agree on the fact that these media products are essentially used as 'poverty porn': voyeuristic entertainment centred on the lives of the poor (Mooney, 2011; Jensen, 2014), and whose most evident effect is the hostile and moralising sentiments against the new undeserving poor that are increasingly unleashed on and legitimised among the public. Take TV shows like *Benefits Street* and *On Benefits and Proud* (Channel 5, 2013). These programmes encapsulate the central features of the moralising discourse against the 'undeserving poor' that emerge in times of moral panic, as defined by Cohen (1972 [2002]: 1). First and foremost, a person or group of persons being identified as a 'threat' to 'societal values and interest'; in this particular case these are the benefit scroungers and their way of life. In these shows people living on benefits are most frequently portrayed as lazy and opportunistic (if not proper cheats) who live beyond their means, spending their benefit money on manicures, alcohol and new TV sets, and are eligible to live in apartments that 'many taxpayers may only dream about', as the voiceover underlines.[14] Secondly, the nature of these people is presented 'in a stylised and stereotypical fashion', is in the case of mother-of-11 Heather Frost, best known to the public of *On Benefits and Proud* as the 'Dole Queen' and 'shameless super scrounger',[15] a title that immediately harks back to the American 'welfare queen'.

It goes without saying that not only do these media products reproduce the moralising and stigmatising discourse against certain categories of poor but they also exacerbate the divisive 'deserving vs undeserving' poor dichotomy in public discourse. TV programmes such as *Saints and Scroungers* (BBC 1, 2009) and *Nick and Margaret: We All Pay Your Benefits* (BBC 1, 2013) are primarily constructed upon the alleged strict opposition between two categories of citizens in terms of values, life conduct and work ethic. *Saints and Scroungers* counterposes the lives of benefits thieves (among whom there are a number of suspected welfare fraudsters) to those of 'people who actually deserve government help',[16] i.e. worthy, often disabled, recipients. Similarly, *We All Pay Your Benefits* relies precisely on the dichotomy narrative, being centred on the encounter of 'honest taxpayers' with unemployed people living on benefits and their expensive lifestyles.

Beyond their voyeuristic intent, most commentators agree, these programmes often contain a strong moral message: that two different categories of poor exist, with a *deviant* group on the one side, being responsible for its own condition and perpetrating an erroneous and 'immoral' way of live; and another one honestly struggling to escape poverty and adhering to social expectations in terms of morale, lifestyle and even 'work ethic' (Huws, 2015). The transposition of the deserving/undeserving poor dichotomy into media representations is by no means a new phenomenon, as the previous sections of this chapter have shown. The parasite/worker hero dichotomy created by communist propaganda in the USSR is a typical example of this mechanism. As was the case in the Soviet experience, the diffusion of 'poverty porn' during the Great Recession cannot be deemed completely accidental. All of the TV programmes mentioned here sprang up between 2009 and 2014, perhaps not incidentally in a period when unemployment levels in the UK reached new heights, rising from 5.2 per cent in 2008 to 8.5 per cent in 2011.[17] This fact is even more striking if we consider how the depiction of poverty and undeserving claimants produced by these TV shows resonates with certain narratives that emerged in the political arena since the inception of the economic crisis, most notably those paralleling an 'anti-welfarism' argument centred on the alleged 'irresponsibility' and moral failure of a part of the British working-class population, referred to as 'Broken Britain' (Mooney, 2011; Hancock and Mooney, 2013).

These political narratives have also insisted on an apparent contrast between two different parts of the British population as the main grounds for discussion when it comes to the British welfare system. Former Chancellor of the Exchequer George Osborne's popular contrast between 'the shift-worker, leaving home in the dark hours of the early morning' and 'their next-door neighbour, sleeping off a life on benefits' became a popular example of the government's emphasis on the distinction between the socially acceptable behaviour of the working class and the deplorable misconduct of able-bodied individuals sponging off the system.[18] However, a new general attitude to the welfare state that rewards the deserving 'striving' worker and penalises, both in symbolic and material terms, the undeserving, 'shirker' claimants has been found to be not the exclusive domain of the Coalition government. The concern expressed by MP Liam Byrne in his speech at the Labour Party Conference in 2011 for the fact that 'many people on the doorstep at the last election felt that too often we were for shirkers not workers' was often repeated, and indicates claims that such a new narrative is found across the political spectrum.

As many commentators have underlined, not only do such distinctions (successfully) attempt to publicly ethically legitimise welfare cuts, something also conveniently used to garner electoral consent from the public, but they also significantly contribute to the emergence of new sentiments of intolerance towards those living on benefits. The recent reported case of death threats made against inhabitants of James Turner Street of *Benefits Street* fame is proof of the growing anger about this very issue.[19] Not surprisingly, in fact, rather than expanding the public's knowledge of poverty and inequality, the spread of 'reality shows' centred on the lives (and lifestyles) of 'undeserving' welfare claimants has ignited an 'anger machine' in UK public opinion, possibly also as the effect of a narrative that often equates welfare claimants and welfare cheats.

However, the return of the old stereotype of the welfare scrounger to the British debate has also been affected by the recent increasing coverage of welfare fraud cases in the popular press, with sensational stories about British welfare scroungers or fraudsters promptly 'validating' the message produced by *Benefits Street* and like-minded TV shows. The number of tabloid pieces dedicated to scroungers and welfare benefits scandals from 2007 to 2015 is notable, with the *Daily Express* and the *Daily Mail* respectively running around 250 different scrounger stories during this period.[20]

Sensationalist headlines such as '75% on sick benefits are faking'[21] or 'Mansions for scroungers: we pay £16m a year to keep families in luxury'[22] have been a mainstay of the popular press since late 2007, with moralising pieces being especially directed at single unemployed mothers on benefits and welfare recipients accused of using the National Health Service (NHS) for plastic surgery, holidays and expensive items.

It may be worth considering at this point whether media coverage of the welfare scrounger debate in Britain comes as a direct effect of the successful broadcast of reality shows such as *Benefits Street* or if the spread of these shows is itself testament to a new dominating attitude towards the undeserving poor among the public. We will explore this topic in the next chapter. Whatever the case however, it can be said that the media amplification of the 'scrounger's life' only provided new material for the 'hard' workfare argument which has by now been at the heart of the UK welfare debate for years and is increasingly gaining ground not only among politicians and commentators but also among the public.

Notes

1 The advent of a 'race to the bottom' scenario predicted by many commentators since the 1970s was essentially based on the argument regarding the 'exhaustion' of the Keynesian welfare state's capacity for further expansion and the alleged incapacity in financial terms to keep pace with the increasing demand for social protection in a capitalist society (O'Connor, 1973; Mishra, 1984). The 'retrenchment' scenario has been put into perspective by Paul Pierson and others, evidencing that the pursuit of political consent represents a major constraint for governments in their attempts at diminishing the welfare state (Pierson, 1994; Pierson, 1996).

2 Callum (1995: 62) reports the draft law distinction between different categories of 'parasites' and their proposed punishment: for 'able-bodied parasites a social sentence of exile' 'could be pronounced [...] (Articles 1–3) [3]; second, vagrants and beggars could be sentenced to the same penalty of exile for a period of between two to five years by a people's court (Article 4); and, third, invalids and the disabled who engaged in vagrancy or begging could be compulsorily confined to special homes for invalids by a decision of the executive committee of the local soviet (Article 5).

3 Law 'For Intensification of the Struggle against Persons Avoiding Socially Useful Work and Leading an Anti-social Parasitic Way of Life' (RSFSR, I961) and former similar laws.

4 *Glasgow Herald*, 14 July 1976.

5 *Lakeland Ledger*, 3 November 1976.

6 *Glasgow Herald*, 5 August 1976.

7 For an in-depth discussion of Lyndon B. Johnson's 'War on Poverty' and successive developments in the history of poor relief programmes in the US see Piven and Cloward (1971); Katz (1983); Katz (1990); Handler and Hasenfeld (1991).

8 A part of the literature has in fact re-examined the argument made by Lewis in his study, and concluded that his anthropological account regarding poverty and subculture has been essentially misinterpreted and used to the advantage of the anti-welfare lobby.

9 '"Welfare Queen' becomes issue in Reagan campaign', *New York Times*, 15 February 1976, p. 51.

10 Handler and Hasenfeld (1991: 113) report that a number of factors – such as social and civil rights activism, the internal migration of African-Americans from Southern states to the North and de-industrialisation and unemployment – contributed to the expansion of this sector of the welfare state, and in particular to the growing inclusion of black unmarried mothers in the system, a prerogative of white mothers until the 1950s. By 1975, '40% of the recipients were white, 44% African-American and 12% Hispanic'.

11 The premiere of the series attracted 4.3 million viewers; data from *The Guardian,* 7 January 2014.

12 Description provided on the BBC webpage of the programme.

13 *The Guardian*, 15 March 2014.

14 Season 1, episode 1.

15 Season 1, episode 1.

16 Description of the programme as available on the BBC show's webpage.

17 Data from the Office for National Statistics, available at www.ons.gov.uk/employment andlabourmarket/peoplenotinwork/unemployment/timeseries/mgsc/unem (accessed 2 October 2016).

18 *The Guardian*, 8 January 2013.

19 *Huffington Post*, 7 January 2014.

20 Author's data collected from journal online databases.

21 *Daily Express*, 14 October 2009.

22 *Daily Express*, 21 February 2010.

6 A new wave of scroungerphobia?

Perceptions of poverty in times of crisis

Introduction

In this chapter we will be exploring the case for the emergence of a new wave of scroungerphobia in Britain. We have previously said that the success of TV programmes such as *Benefits Street* and the increasing coverage of welfare fraud cases in the press are illustrative of the fact that the issue of the undeserving poor has recently reappeared in many countries. One of the main objectives in this book is to analyse the relationship between socio-economic crises and the treatment of the undeserving poor at different points in time and in different contexts. We have already looked at the political treatment of undeserving welfare claimants over time and at the social representations of them produced by the media. We will now explore the territory of public opinion and perception. The central theme of this book is that at different moments in modern times social and economic crises have been accompanied by episodes of 'moral panic', resulting, among other things, in the exacerbation of sentiments of being threatened and general anxiety towards the poor. The exaggerated Victorian preoccupation with the morality of the 'dangerous classes' (Himmelfarb, 1991: 7) is one example of the moral panic that is discussed in this book. The Great Recession of 2007–2009 and its aftermath constitute another interesting time frame to explore for our purposes.

Recent studies on social attitudes during austerity (such as the *British Social Attitudes Report*) have shown that sympathy towards social benefit recipients has decreased in the UK compared to similar periods in the past. Not only has public support in favour of unemployment programmes declined, but the report also brings new evidence to light on existing profound misconceptions concerning welfare issues and related statistics. In 2011, for example, 37 per cent of the British public believed that most welfare recipients 'fiddle', while 35 per cent stated that social security payments frequently go to those who 'don't really deserve any help' (Clery, 2012: 11). Likewise, a Trades Union Congress (TUC) poll published in 2013 revealed that the UK public generally believes that 41 per cent of all British welfare spending goes to the unemployed, as opposed to the much lower actual figure (3 per cent), and that on average people believe that 27 per cent of the UK welfare budget is *fraudulently claimed*, while the real percentage is 0.7 per cent.[1]

These findings are of particular importance to our study as they shed light on how *misconceptions* and misunderstanding regarding the welfare state may generate negative sentiments and opinions towards those considered undeserving of social support. An example can help clarify this process. Another important misconception concerning the welfare state which is poignantly described in a recent study by John Hills (2015: 23) is that the 'poor are too expensive' for our society, an argument, Hills evidences, which parallels the decreasing support among the British population for *welfare benefits* as a component of the social budget since the mid-1990s, and possibly also for *redistribution* as a function of the welfare state.

Having clarified that there is a direct link between misconceptions about the welfare state and attitudes towards claimants and benefits, it is therefore worth further investigating the realm of public perceptions and opinion, and whether the recent crisis and wave of austerity measures have been paralleled not only by increasing misconceptions about the welfare state but also by the emergence of *anti-scrounger* sentiments. Our discussion will consist of two parts. In the first part of this chapter we will look at attitudes towards poverty during the Great Recession. Drawing upon data from the Eurobarometer on the UK case, we will discuss the transformation of attitudes to poverty and the poor during the years of the crisis (2007–2010). Then the second part will explore sentiments about deservedness in the British welfare state in more depth. Original results from a focus group study conducted in the post-recession context (2015–2016) will be presented and discussed.

It is important to clarify that the following study focuses solely on the British case for a number of reasons. Firstly, a widespread public debate exists in the UK on the topics examined here which is unparalleled in most European countries. At the same time, the diffusion of media entertainment products centred on the lives of welfare recipients is unprecedented in Britain (see Chapter 5), making the UK case a unique testing ground for the analysis we intend to pursue in this chapter. Moreover, as will be clarified below, the UK constitutes an interesting exception in Europe that is worth considering for the purposes of our work.

Interpretations of poverty in times of economic crisis

Any analysis that aims at studying attitudes to deservedness in the welfare state should start from Serge Paugam's milestone work on contemporary perceptions of poverty in Europe. A central conclusion in his study is that, despite great 'structural' variation across countries (i.e. perceptions on poverty change across space), collective attitudes towards the poor are profoundly marked by a 'conjecture effect' (perceptions change over time) (Paugam and Selz, 2005: 292; Paugam, 2009). More specifically, in times of crisis (for example when unemployment grows) the conjecture effect would tend to make people more inclined to understand and describe poverty in terms of social injustice and more reluctant to explain it as an effect of idleness and individual failure. While this might be true for attitudes to poverty in general, as in Paugam's analysis, it is certainly less evident when one considers narratives focusing on a specific category of poor, the undeserving poor. However, the argument made here – that latent sentiments against the undeserving poor can be exacerbated in times of 'moral crisis' – does not necessarily contrast with Paugam's finding that crises can prompt solidaristic attitudes towards the poor. Paugam himself recognises that in some countries, most notably the UK, interpretations of poverty based on idleness can become prevalent, especially in conjunction with economic crisis. Based on this result, we can examine the British exception in depth by discussing it during and after the recent international crisis.

From a theoretical point of view, our analysis is based upon the classification proposed by Clarke and Cochrane (1998: 14, 16), who identify three major distinct normative orientations guiding common-sense ideas about poverty as a social problem and the main explanations given for it:

- Attitudes that understand poverty as a 'natural and inevitable' phenomenon, even 'socially necessary' to encourage individuals to succeed, in what we could refer to as a competition for the survival of the fittest. This attitude could be termed *functionalist*.
- Attitudes that perceive poverty as a condition produced by the specific character or behaviour of the poor. We can define common sense beliefs deriving from such an approach as *culturalistic* after the well-known theory of Oscar Lewis (1959) on the 'culture of poverty'. These attitudes assign a predominant role to individual flaws and alleged deviant behaviour in determining poverty.
- *Social* interpretations of poverty, which view this phenomenon as the 'effect of economic or political causes'. Such an approach views poverty as mainly determined by social structures that are 'outside the individual's control'.
- This third classification can be supplemented by a fourth category, comprising *fatalistic* attitudes towards poverty, i.e. orientations driven by the understanding of poverty as an inevitable and unfortunate event.

Against this background, we can examine whether the inception of the economic crisis in the UK altered the perception of poverty among the British population. Drawing upon this classification, we can easily apply Eurobarometer data from 2007, 2009 and 2010 to the four above-mentioned interpretative typologies.

Returning to 2007, before the inception of the international crisis, Eurobarometer data for the UK reveal that, when asked the question 'Why in your opinion are there people who live in need?', the majority of British respondents provided a *culturalistic* explanation for the existence of poverty,

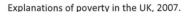

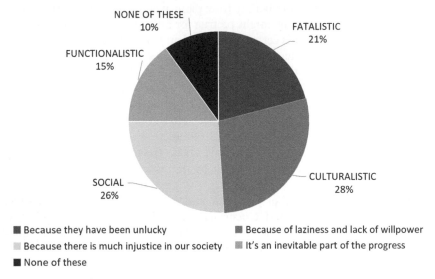

Figure 6.1 Explanations of poverty in the UK, 2007
Source: Author's calculation from Eurobarometer data (Eurobarometer 67.1, 'Cultural values, poverty and social exclusion, developmental aid, and residential mobility', February–March 2007) based on the classification of Clarke and Cochrane (1998).

indicating 'laziness and lack of willpower' as the main explanations for this phenomenon (Figure 6.1). A few years into the economic crisis, in 2009, interpretations of poverty in the UK became much more associated with a *social* explanation. As Figure 6.2 illustrates, the proportion of persons providing a culturalistic interpretation of poverty remained high even during the peak (2008–2009) of the global crisis that brought Britain into its deepest recession since World War II (Brewer et al., 2013).

However, on this occasion a much greater proportion of respondents viewed poverty and need as conditions essentially derived from 'injustice in our society'. After the peak of the recession in 2010, and in conjunction with a slow recovery from the crisis, culturalistic interpretations of poverty began losing ground (Figure 6.3). At the same time, interestingly, the proportion of respondents who provided a functionalistic explanation for poverty (seen as an 'inevitable part of progress') increased significantly as compared to 2007 and 2009. These results are not at variance with Paugam's argument that solidaristic interpretations of poverty increase in times of crisis. They do, however, indicate the exceptionality of the UK case where a culturalistic interpretation of poverty was predominant even before 2007. It is important, in fact, to point out that the proportion of people who offered a culturalistic explanation of poverty did not decrease (in fact it grew slightly) even during the peak of the recession. This is especially evident if we consider that even at a time when unemployment reached its highest levels during the recession,

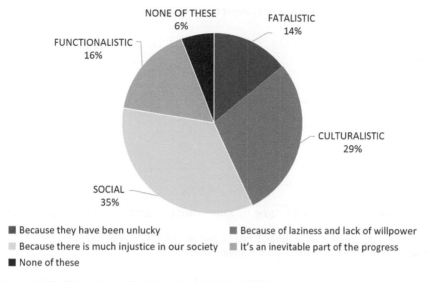

Figure 6.2 Explanations of poverty in the UK, 2009
Source: Author's calculation from Eurobarometer data (Special Eurobarometer 321: 'Poverty and social exclusion; wave 72.1: poverty and social exclusion, social services, climate change, and the national economic situation and statistics', August–September 2009) based on the classification of Clarke and Cochrane (1998).

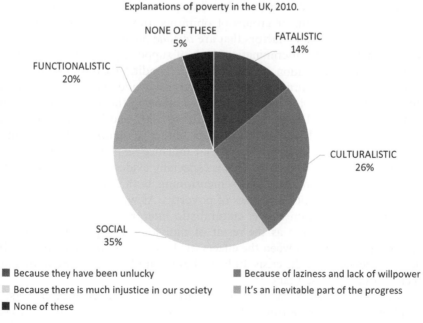

Figure 6.3 Explanations of poverty in the UK, 2010
Source: Author's calculation from Eurobarometer data (Special Eurobarometer 74.1: Poverty and Social Exclusion, Mobile Phone Use, Economic Crisis, and International Trade, August–September 2010) based on the classification of Clarke and Cochrane (1998).

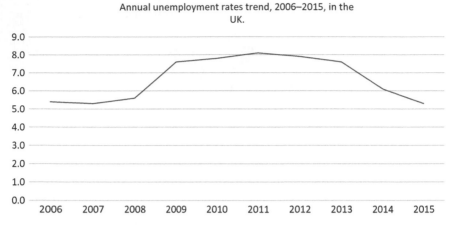

Figure 6.4 Unemployment annual rates trend in the UK, 2006–2015
Source: Author's calculation from Eurostat database.

almost a third of the respondents viewed poverty as caused by laziness and lack of willpower (Figure 6.4).

The distinctive, reverse 'conjuncture effect' of the crisis on the UK case, however, is much more manifest when we look at how people interpret poverty in terms of *personal factors* that might explain this phenomenon. Based on data for the question 'Which three of the following reasons might best explain why people are poor or excluded from our society?', the answers may be divided into two major groups of opinions: those identifying poverty as predominantly created by factors that are *outside the individual's control* (such as low social benefits, discrimination, lack of support, poor health) and those based on an identification of poverty as a condition caused by *individual failure* (addiction to drugs or alcohol, living beyond one's means, lack of education and having too many children). Following this distinction, we have grouped and analysed answers collected during 2007 and 2010. Interpretations of poverty which rely on the 'individual failure' assumption became much more pronounced as compared to 'social injustice' explanations (Figures 6.5 and 6.6) during 2007 and 2010. This is especially evident when we look at the significant increase in respondents mentioning both 'living beyond means' and 'educational deficits' as causes of poverty.[2] As was the case with the first Eurobarometer question above, culturalistic interpretations of poverty connoting this phenomenon as the result of individual (supposedly wrong) life decisions persisted even when the effects of the recession became more visible with the deepening of the crisis. In fact, these attitudes became more frequent precisely during those years.

These data seem consistent with Paugam's idea of the British case as an exception to the 'solidaristic' effect on attitudes that is generally observed in times of crisis. This is not to say of course that solidarity does not exist in Britain, but rather is an indication of the fact that culturalistic interpretations

CAUSES OF POVERTY, OPINIONS, UK, 2007

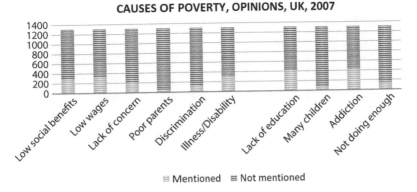

☰ Mentioned ☰ Not mentioned

Figure 6.5 Causes of poverty in the UK, 2007
Source: Author's calculation from Eurobarometer data (Eurobarometer 67.1: 'Cultural values, poverty and social exclusion, developmental aid, and residential mobility', February–March 2007).

CAUSES OF POVERTY, OPINIONS, UK, 2009

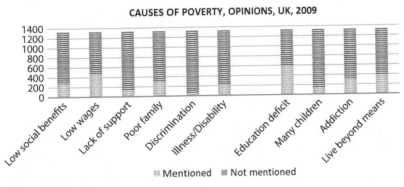

☰ Mentioned ☰ Not mentioned

Figure 6.6 Causes of poverty in the UK, 2009
Author's calculation from Eurobarometer data (Special Eurobarometer 321: 'Poverty and social exclusion; wave 72.1: poverty and social exclusion, social services, climate change, and the national economic situation and statistics', August–September 2009).

of poverty persist there even in times of crisis. Recession and austerity may even aggravate negative attitudes to the 'idle' poor, not least as an indirect effect of political and media narratives. The press coverage of welfare fraud cases, as we said, may have a decisive role in spreading a distorted perception of the extent of the phenomenon among the public. At the same time, political rhetoric appealing to the 'unsustainable' cost of social policy programmes for Britain as a justification for welfare cuts may re-enforce negative attitudes for 'undeserving' claimants.[3]

Having briefly discussed data from the Eurobarometer, it is now evident that they can only provide an overview of general attitudes towards poverty and its main causes. In order to further understand sentiments and opinions

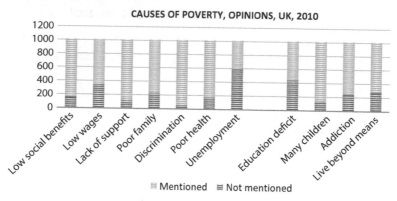

CAUSES OF POVERTY, OPINIONS, UK, 2010

⊟ Mentioned   ≡ Not mentioned

Figure 6.7 Causes of poverty in the UK, 2010
Source: Author's calculation from Eurobarometer data (Special Eurobarometer 74.1: 'Poverty and social exclusion, mobile phone use, economic crisis, and international trade', August–September 2010).

about the welfare state and 'deserving' categories in times of crisis we must necessarily refer to information obtained with qualitative methods. A focus group analysis centred on these themes can complement our discussion and provide further insights into how individuals construct their interpretative frameworks around the notion of deservedness in the welfare state.

The background to the 'Rhonda experiment'

An important study by Petersen et al. has illustrated that, when questioned on welfare issues, individuals react not only by responding according to their political values but also and predominantly by resorting to their 'deserving-ness heuristic', which is a cognitive framework made of decision rules that 'prompts citizens to consider whether recipients deserve their welfare benefits and premise their opinion on this evaluation' (2010: 26). According to the authors, an important element in the formulation of perceptions, and parti-cularly of an individual's deservingness heuristic, is the sort of *information* each person receives concerning a given recipient or welfare scheme. How the media portray the poor or specific categories of welfare claimants, for example, may significantly impact a person's deservedness framework, thus also affecting his or her immediate views and opinions about the welfare system. The role of the media in constructing a social perception of undeserving poor is therefore an important point of departure in any study that aims at investigating deservingness categories, attitudes to notions of social justice, equality and merit in the welfare state and their application to reality.

It is also the point of departure of another important work, the 'welfare queen' experimental study conducted by American political scientist Franklin D. Gilliam (1999). The study aimed at showing that the welfare queen myth that emerged in the 1960s had become a 'narrative script' in the US by the end of the century, meaning it had acquired the status of 'common knowledge' among the public. Gilliam's idea for the study drew upon two of the predominant media narratives (or stereotypes) about the welfare system in the US: a) that most welfare recipients are *women*, and b) that most women on welfare are *African-American*. Having identified 'gender' and 'race' as the two predominant components of media discourse on welfare, Gilliam conducted a visual experiment in 1999 on a group of people watching television news. Viewers were asked to watch videotaped TV news on the invented but realistic story of Rhonda Germaine, a woman concerned for her and her children's future based on an anticipated welfare reforms. Each group of participants watched one of three different videotapes, with the first one portraying Rhonda as a white woman, the second one casting a black Rhonda and the third one with no picture of Rhonda. A fourth set of respondents who watched no TV story at all served as the control group. A post-test questionnaire was then given to all participants, exploring their views on welfare, race and gender, and in particular disclosing attitudes concerning causes and solutions to welfare as an issue, attitudes on racial stereotypes and beliefs about gender roles. One of the most interesting findings of the study is that the representation of the 'quintessential welfare queen' (i.e. the black Rhonda) did not elicit as much anti-black sentiment among the viewers as the exposure to the white Rhonda did; but it did provoke strong anti-welfare opinions among these respondents, who, incidentally, would refer to individual failure as the main cause of poverty and social issues in general.

Our study: objectives and method

The Rhonda experiment is a pioneering work in the study of how media representations of the undeserving poor impact the audience's views on the welfare system as a whole. In this part of the chapter we will analyse the results of a study that we have conducted by using Gilliam's experiment as the main background study and with the main purpose being to investigate the relations between media perceptions and opinions on the contemporary welfare 'scrounger' in the UK.

The study was held during 2015 and 2016, comprising four different focus group meetings conducted in London, with groups consisting of approximately 8–10 participants per session. The study had two main objectives. The first was to explore the role of the media in producing a social perception of the undeserving poor in times of crisis and its potential impact on opinions and beliefs concerning the welfare state. The second was to identify the main categories of deservedness among the public and to assess the case for a new wave of 'scroungerphobia' in the UK. The main rationale for the study was provided by the increasing coverage of welfare fraud and welfare benefit scandal stories in the British press in recent years, and especially since the onset of the Great Recession (2007–2008), coupled with the great success of 'poverty entertainment' products such as *Benefits Street* and similar TV shows. As in the case for the Rhonda experiment, our study starts by identifying the predominant components of British media narratives on the undeserving poor. Both channels of information, the popular press and TV shows, have nurtured a number of specific stereotypes over the years, most of which refer to the existence of allegedly recurrent types of 'undeserving claimants', notably single mothers, the false disabled, unworthy immigrants and the very archetype of all undeserving poor, the idle unemployed.

A focus group technique – i.e. interviews with different groups of respondents – was selected as the most appropriate research method for the study. Evidence from the literature has validated the use of focus group discussions as one of the best methods for eliciting opinions, attitudes and beliefs from respondents in an informal environment (Carey and Asbury, 2012). Focus groups have been defined as 'performances in which the participants jointly produce accounts about proposed topics' (Smithson, 2008: 363) or as 'invaluable' instruments that provide 'insights into how *meaning is constructed*' (Kamberelis and Dimitriadis, 2013: 11, emphasis added). The latter element is of particular importance for the purpose of our analysis, which is directed at understanding how attitudes towards the undeserving poor are actually constructed. Most prominently, research that aims at identifying ideas of deservedness and ethical frameworks concerning social justice among the public may respond very well to focus group discussions wherein respondents may feel more comfortable to freely express their views and opinions on a particular matter, as opposed to traditional face-to-face interviews. Moreover, debate among participants may well provoke discussion that expands on unexpected topics or matters of significant importance for the study but not necessarily mentioned in the focus group script.

Participants for all our focus groups were recruited online through online advertisements, and were offered a small cash compensation (£10) plus a travel refund. Each group discussion was organised in three different parts with an overall duration of two hours per session. A topic list which included both main questions and probes was written and used for all meetings. Following a brief introduction about the aims and general content of the research, participants were asked to introduce themselves. During the three rounds of questions, a number of issues were posed by the focus group moderator, covering different aspects of welfare state claimants; the ideal role of the welfare state; its main failures and benefits; priorities in the social protection system; categories of claimants that should be protected at all costs in a society; and groups (if any) that should be excluded from social redistribution are some examples of the issues touched on during each meeting.

Around 60 minutes into the discussion, participants were divided into two groups. A photocopy of a tabloid article featuring a real benefits scandal story was then distributed separately to group A and group B. The piece discussed the *true* story of a woman who pleaded guilty to charges of having gathered thousands of pounds from a benefits fraud after her entitlement to the benefits – paid on the basis that she was unemployed, single and living alone with three children – dissolved when she went to live with her husband, failing to inform the authorities. The article distributed to group A featured the real name of the fraudster, an English woman from the north-west of the country, and her picture, which portrayed her as white and blonde. Group B received the same article, the only difference being the name of the person, which was substituted with a Central/Eastern Europe-sounding name of another existing fraudster in the UK and her picture, depicting a Central/Eastern European woman with a scarf covering her head. Still separately, the two groups were asked to read the story and to comment on the case featured in the article and to define the content of the story. Furthermore, they were asked how frequent and typical they thought cases like the one in the article were in the UK, and to further expand on the causes and motivation for the welfare fraud story they read. All participants then gathered in one meeting room for a final discussion where opinions were elicited again on a number of issues posed at the beginning of the focus group section.

Analysis and main findings

The four focus groups were recorded with a digital voice recorder and transcribed. Then all transcripts were analysed to explore different themes and issues of the study. Special attention was devoted to analysing the experimental session and to comparing the findings from the two different groups of participants. Finally, a word cloud technique was used to provide a visual representation of the main results of the study.[4]

A total of 38 people took part in the focus groups (14 men and 24 women). All participants had no professional-based knowledge of the British welfare system, and mainly derived their opinions and beliefs from common sense, personal experiences and public sources of information – e.g. newspapers, TV and the internet. Results from the focus group meetings may be discussed from the perspective of three main themes or dimensions addressing stereotypical representations of welfare claimants: the *deserving/undeserving categorisation* and the *media effect* respectively.

Stereotypical welfare claimant representations

The first question addressed to all participants in the focus group was: What is the first thing that comes to your mind when hearing the word 'welfare'? Participants were asked to answer the question promptly based either on their own experience, opinions, beliefs or information from the media. A word cloud graph summarising the most recurrent words and concepts associated with the term 'welfare' during the meetings is provided in Figure 6.8. We predicted that most of the participants' imagery would reproduce part of the stereotypical representations produced by the media and by dominant political views on the welfare state. A common element emerging from the discussion is that, when elicited on this topic, most of the participants tended to separate

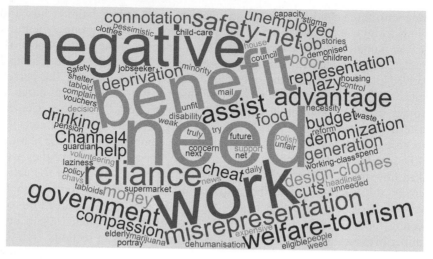

Figure 6.8 Word cloud representation of associations with the term 'welfare'
Source: Author's elaboration from own data.

their *own ideas* from those constructed by the media and political *narratives*. More specifically, many participants recognised that part of the images in their minds when thinking about the word 'welfare' were not so much linked to real experiences and personal knowledge on the matter, but often rather to stories and debates about welfare claimants circulating in the media. Overall reactions to this question may be divided into two main groups.

One group of respondents reported that the media have a strong impact on the (negative) representation of welfare recipients, and underlined the role played both by press coverage and politicians alike in re-enforcing these stereotypes. Many of these respondents acknowledged that these portrayals were generally unfair to the majority of those in a true condition of need, and condemned them for their potential detrimental psychological effects on the recipient population. However, most participants contemplated the risk of people 'taking advantage' of their welfare state, with claimants cheating or exploiting the system 'even if they do not need it' being the general rule. When thinking about the word 'welfare', many participants immediately mentioned examples of family or friends using their benefits to buy alcohol, drugs or luxury items such as designer clothes or upgraded TV sets.

Another group associated the word 'welfare' with feelings of pessimism and scepticism, basing their sentiments predominantly on their own understanding of the social protection system. Most frequently, among the spontaneous causes for concern expressed by participants on this topic was the uncertain *sustainability* of the present system for future generations; the lack of compassion from the public on the stigmatisation of persons who cannot possibly work (most notably the disabled); and the departure of the welfare system from its original intent of providing 'wellbeing' to its citizens. Furthermore, a majority of the group immediately associated the term 'welfare' with the ongoing cuts in the social protection system. Among those who approved of the idea of reforms, many referred to the need to change a system apparently too generous for certain categories, such as immigrants. Welfare 'tourism' – i.e. the arrival of immigrants in the country for the sole purpose of accessing welfare benefits and free health care – was mentioned very often and was especially discussed in conjunction with concerns about the inadequate checks by the institutions on eligibility, regulations regarding conditions and sanctions, and about the increasing cases of benefit *fraud*.

Overall, the welfare perception of participants was dominated by pessimism and negative views of the current system. With few exceptions, most participants associated the word 'welfare' essentially with the *social benefit* system and in particular with *cash transfers*. Only on a few occasions did participants mention social security, pension schemes and the tax credit system for workers. Predominantly, participants imagined welfare as cash payments for those in a condition of 'need', as a 'safety net' to help those who have lost their jobs, are unqualified to find another one or are unfit to perform working activities.

When asked for their opinions about what is the *most typical category* of welfare claimant in the UK, the majority of participants answered that lone mothers, the unemployed, the elderly and the disabled are the most common category of recipient in their country. However, when asked to expand on their thoughts on this topic, many persons in the group referred to the fact that not only the 'truly poor' access the welfare system, and that it is very common for 'scroungers', 'false depressed', 'obese' persons to easily 'fiddle' the system and access welfare benefits. On this topic however, while a number of participants insisted that this is only a perception driven by press coverage and political narratives, the most common sentiment was that of blaming both the system for its loopholes and the individual for taking advantage of common resources that should be transferred to those in a real condition of need. The analysis of this first dimension tends to confirm the certain impact of dominant stereotypes and narratives in public opinion, and in particular the construction of the social representation of the welfare claimant in our society. Among all of the dimensions taken into consideration, certain media portrayals such as those produced by *Benefits Street* proved to have a stronger impact on respondents as compared to political narratives. Quite often 'welfare scrounger' definitions provided by participants invoked concepts from these very TV shows or tabloid headlines. Contrary to our expectations, only to a lesser extent were dominant narratives produced in the political arena conducive to the construction of specific representations of welfare and welfare claimants.

Deserving vs undeserving claimants

Another theme that we explored in the analysis of our focus group was the 'deservingness heuristic' (Petersen et al., 2010). We attempted to understand how each participant gives shape to his/her framework that regulates the answer to the underlying question: 'Who deserves to be helped in our society?' We also tried to understand how these frameworks are constructed. Are they morally driven? Are they affected by each person's direct experience? Are they imbued by political or religious beliefs? These questions were all taken into account not only by analysing the direct answers of each participant to the themes posed by the moderator, but also by looking at the interaction between participants in each focus group. Most frequently we found that the strongest opinions and beliefs about deservedness were expressed by participants when disagreeing or agreeing with others' arguments.

A first set of answers analysed are those to the question: 'Should you have the opportunity to be in charge of the welfare budget and could decide based on your personal preferences, what welfare programme/category would you give priority to?' We expected that participants' answers would mostly be affected by the dominant media and political narratives. Answers to this question however varied significantly. Overall, the majority of the discussion over priorities in the welfare state – and indirectly the one over deservingness – was dominated by two main dimensions. The most visible element in all the discussions made in our focus groups was the *ability/disability* issue. When asked to 'save' just one sector of the welfare state, most participants identified support for disabled people as the welfare compartment that should be protected at any cost by collectivity. This choice was formulated mostly by means of fatalistic explanations: those with a physical handicap or deficiency cannot be *blamed* and punished for being unfit to work and must be helped by society. At a general level, most arguments in defence of the disabled as a 'deserving' category were re-enforced with arguments against able-bodied individuals who can work but are unwilling to do so. Contrary to our expectations, reference to the 'false' disabled debate was very seldom made by participants, and in most of the cases only to express concern for the impact of the *Work Capability Assessment*, both in terms of the stigmatisation of claimants and the economic consequences they face when losing their benefits.

This brings us to another important component in the discussion: the 'work ethic' dimension. The argument against providing generous welfare payments to those who can but do not work often emerged in the discussion, proving that individual *willingness to work* is the first and most important criterion needed to evaluate whether a person should be deserving or not of social protection. Many in the group explicitly referred to the need to reform job centres as a priority, so that money directed at those who cannot find a job despite looking for it may be provided with help. This argument was often paralleled by concerns about the lack of adequate incentives to work on the part of the bureaucratic system. Moreover, the work ethic dimension issue was raised in the group almost every time the *immigration* topic was posed. We anticipated this topic to be felt as a thorny issue during the discussion, and that participants might have been reluctant to express strong views and opinions against immigrants as a deserving category. Contrary to these expectations however, most people expressed criticism of how the British welfare system rewards (especially non-labouring) immigrants in the country, basing this view predominantly on the argument that at the same time many 'honest' British taxpayers are often unable to make ends meet as a consequence of ongoing welfare cuts.

It is worth noting that in all of the focus group discussions that we conducted the topic of immigrants as an undeserving category of welfare claimant emerged at some point. In fact, immigrants were never mentioned as a 'deserving' category (or a priority) by participants, while the topic of European and non-EU immigrants accessing welfare benefits was commonly raised also when discussing the main problems of the British welfare state. 'Polish', 'Romanian' and 'Central/Eastern European' were mostly referred to during such discussions. 'Asylum seekers' were also mentioned on some occasions as categories that should be excluded from all sorts of welfare redistribution, and more frequently during the fourth focus group (January 2016), when the refugee crisis in Europe assumed increasing visibility in the press and in public debate.

Another important perspective was ideology and political views regarding deservedness. When imagining their 'ideal welfare state', many participants insisted that their opinions were based on certain ideological or political beliefs. For example, when formulating the concept that an ideal welfare state should favour a redistribution from the 'haves' to the 'have-nots', one of the participants clarified that this opinion was essentially driven by her 'communist-oriented' view of the world. In other cases, participants justified their deserv-ingness frameworks by explicitly mentioning politicians' speeches or campaigns from the right wing. Predominantly, official views of parties such as UKIP were not approved of in the group, but it was not uncommon for participants to approve of some of their 'Euroscepticism' which was mentioned, again when immigration and welfare tourism was taken into account along with the 'deservedness' topic.

Finally, a further dimension of deservedness emerging from this part of the discussion was the *vulnerability* factor. Together with the disabled and veterans, children were often felt to be the most immediate category needing indisputable protection by society. The emotional dimension in the construction of a deservingness heuristic can be said to be stronger in most of the focus groups conducted. However, mixed feelings emerged when specific categories were considered. When the case of lone mothers with many children was discussed in the group, for example, the emotional dimension was often found to be abandoned for moralistic explanations. While admitting that children had to be protected, it was not uncommon for participants to be highly critical of lone mothers who are dependent on welfare payments, especially if they have multiple children. The most frequent explanation for this – which comes from both men and women in the group – is essentially *moralistic*: the behaviour of a mother who gives birth to many children when she cannot properly feed them is felt by many participants as something that should not be economically incentivised by the state. It is interesting to note that children thus fall into two different categories, depending on the classification of the mother as a deserving or undeserving claimant.

Overall, it can be said that the deservingness heuristics of our participants responded both to individual rationales (i.e. moralistic, emotional or ideological ones) and to collective concepts and dominant narratives regarding deserving/undeserving categories of claimants. Interestingly, there were a number of topics that proved to be more sensitive to individual normative and ideological frameworks (such as the idea that disabled persons and children should always receive social support) and other issues more receptive of the narratives made in the public debate – most notably those emerging in response to the question of whether immigrants should deserve social protection or not. These frameworks were often found to parallel the argument made by politicians in defence of cuts to the welfare state, and only to a lower degree to respond to personal opinions made on ideological or moralistic grounds.

The media effect

The purpose of Gilliam's study was to investigate the case for the promotion in US public opinion of welfare queen stereotypes regarding race and gender. Similarly, we used an experimental approach in the third part of our focus group study to understand the effects of news stories that validate or, conversely, contrast the ideas generally transmitted by the media. Having randomly divided each group into two subgroups (group A and group B) we collected their answers and analysed our transcripts to identify participants' reactions to the two stories. We predicted that those in group B would express stronger opinions against the welfare system compared to those in group A, based on the fact that the visual representation of the 'Romanian' benefit fraud (group B) would serve as a *validation* of the widespread view of immigrants as undeserving claimants and 'common' cheats. Likewise, we anticipated that the fraud case with the subject depicted as an English white woman (group A) would trigger mixed sentiments of condemnation and justification.

During the discussion and the analysis of the focus group experiment transcripts, two predominant patterns became evident. Firstly, reactions to the 'white woman' story showed only a little surprise among participants. Most of those in the room commented on the story that it was 'most common' in the UK and labelled the story as 'just another exaggerated headline for a benefit fraud case' but not necessarily a 'crime'. The woman was generally described as a 'normal' person subject to the 'name and shame' procedure in the popular press for the sake of sensationalism. Most of those in group A agreed that it was too harsh a treatment and representation of this particular woman given the 'small amount' of money that she had illicitly obtained.

Similarly, in group B most participants immediately identified the story as a common case of fraud, and there were mixed reactions regarding whether this could be labelled as a proper case of crime or not. However, when asked to expand on their views on the newspaper case and to attempt to explain the *factors* behind the story, differences between the two groups became more evident.

Some of the participants in group A indicated problems with alcohol, drugs or an abusive husband among the potential factors explaining the woman's behaviour, while others blamed her lack of *responsibility* in financial terms and possibly her incapacity to distinguish 'between right and wrong'. Part of this last group insisted that she might have found herself in a 'financial trap' and suggested that cases like hers are typical of the underclass and people living at the margins of our society in general. Many also felt that this particular sort of news story is in fact responsible for the spread of negative stereotypes of welfare claimants among the public.

In any case, this opinion was not shared by everyone. In fact, some in the group labelled the story as a typical case of 'middle-class crime' that is generally neglected by the popular press. Interestingly, no other context concerning the socio-economic background of the woman was given to participants, thus we can imagine that her middle-class status was mainly assumed based on visual representation of the woman and the name provided in the article. Only on a few occasions did some of the participants mention the lack of control over welfare claimants as a factor behind cases like these.

Explanations of the case featured in story B revealed a different dynamic. Many agreed that it might be just a common case of a 'mother in need'. Female participants in the group in particular showed a certain sympathy for the woman and said they could certainly relate to the situation of a struggling mother in a foreign country who failed to inform the authorities that her living arrangements had (possibly temporarily) changed. However, the majority of participants, both men and women, agreed on the fact that a major factor in the case reported is the inefficient system of *control* in the welfare system. Many in group B believed that dishonest people trying to cheat the welfare system exist both among immigrants and natives, and that it is only thanks to the loopholes in the bureaucratic mechanisms of control and sanctions that people can easily get away with fraud.

'Greed' was a common answer participants gave when asked for the reasons that might have led the woman to act in such a way. Whether a crime or not, the majority of participants believed that a fraud was committed in attempting to 'maximise' the amount of the benefit and to earn more money. However, and unlike reactions to story A, the discussion in group B was often dominated by the feeling that this particular woman should be 'rightfully' punished and possibly sent back to her country. When compared with reactions to story A, explanations provided by participants for the 'Central/Eastern Europe case' evidenced that the fraud she committed was generally perceived by participants as more severe a crime. Tolerance of the British government towards welfare tourism cases was mentioned as one of the predominant causes for the worsening situation in the country, and some believed that the woman might well have been part of an international criminal organisation 'fiddling' the system from abroad.

Concluding remarks

Looking at the four focus groups conducted, it is possible to summarise all findings by identifying two main differences, predominantly found between the two groups of participants in our experiment. Group A largely attributed an 'individual failure' to the woman depicted in the news. Criminal intent or exploitation of the loopholes in the welfare system were only partially touched on as issues during the meetings. Most of those in group A recognised that the woman was guilty but explained her wrongdoing predominantly in terms of bad *personal choices*.

Conversely, discussions in group B were mostly dominated by the argument that the British welfare state is too generous or lax in controlling welfare recipients. The story of the 'Romanian' woman was rarely discussed as a case of personal shortcoming or individual failure. In the end, one principal, solid difference can be identified between the two sets of participants, with those from group A expressing concerns for the *moral* shortcomings of welfare fraudsters and often attributing this behaviour to *cultural* reasons (e.g. the idea that people from the underclass might be incapable of 'distinguishing between right and wrong'), and those in group B revealing anxieties about the *economic exploitation* of the British welfare system by immigrants, both European and non-EU.

In the light of the original intentions and questions of our study, a number of conclusions can be drawn. Firstly, these results allow us to better understand the role of the media and political narratives in the construction of deservingness heuristics among the public. Contrary to some of our predictions, our findings suggest that personal views and opinions generally underlie the majority of arguments made in support of a certain category of deserving claimant, which means that, generally speaking, respondents' answers seem to rely on individual experience or on ethical or ideological preferences.

However, a number of topics prove to be particularly sensitive to the *dominant* stereotypes and narratives played out in the public sphere. Among these, immigration as an issue and the question of whether immigrants, refugees and asylum seekers should be considered deserving of social protection are often associated with politicians' campaigns or declarations. In many cases this theme evokes prompt reference to stories read in the news. The question of whether immigrants are a deserving or undeserving category is at the centre of all discussion on the deficiencies of the British welfare state and its budget. Furthermore, views on the 'expensive living standards' of certain categories of welfare claimants often evoked images or stereotypical representations made both in the press and on TV.

An unpredicted result however is the common acknowledgement by all groups that public perceptions of welfare claimants in the UK are profoundly shaped by media portrayals. Participants are not unaware of the role of the media in constructing a certain kind of representation of 'undeserving' claimants, and often attribute the emphasis given to stories of welfare fraud to a specific attempt at reinforcing politicians' campaigns in defence of welfare cuts.

It is more challenging to answer the most important of our initial questions, which is whether or not public anxiety about welfare fraud cases has assumed the proportion of a new wave of scroungerphobia. This question can only be addressed by also looking at the 'experimental' phase of our study. If we dealt only with the general discussion made in the first part of our focus groups, we could easily conclude that the debate is by no means suggestive of a scroungerphobia sentiment among participants. Most people in the groups, as noted in fact, do disapprove of the narratives that are critical of the 'undeserving' poor made in newspapers and TV shows, and express strong criticism of the stigmatising impact that they can have on claimants. However, if we analyse the findings from the experimental part of our study, it is indisputable that to a great extent there is general anxiety and concern among participants. Of the two stories it is mostly the 'Romanian' case that prompts the strongest reactions. Although no indication is given in the article that the woman is in fact a foreign citizen, all participants in group B assumed that she must not be a British national, supposedly basing this belief on the visual content and name provided in the news. The interiorisation of the public debate against immigrants taking advantage of the British welfare state can be thus identified as a first general conclusion. Even without details contextualising the fraud story, most discussions in group B are led by the fear that immigrants can take advantage of British resources.

In a parallel way, discussion in group A is also suggestive of sentiments of concern for the sustainability of the welfare system vis-à-vis the lack of control, but this occurs only to a much lower extent as compared to the 'immigrant' case. This too mainly refers to the risk of a 'moral' breakdown of the population rather than its potential economic consequences. In conclusion, it can be said that if an interiorisation of dominant representations of undeserving claimants has occurred in the aftermath of the Great Recession, this has predominantly concerned the view of immigrants as a potential economic threat to collective resources, i.e. the British welfare state, especially at a time when the national budget is under continuous review.

This sentiment has not substituted moralising attacks aimed at those deemed undeserving of social protection, as the discussion in group A of our focus group has suggested. The 'white English woman' case, after all, also validates a stereotype – and precisely the one based on the idea that lone mothers with many children fall into the category of 'undeserving' claimants since they irresponsibly give birth to children that they cannot raise without being 'dependent' on the welfare system. A further significant factor in this discussion is the continuous parallel presence of moral and economic rationales for the justification of deservedness heuristics among the public. However, and in line with the previous chapter, these findings are consistent with the idea that anxiety about the 'economic' threat to collective resources is increasingly substituting sentiments of concerns about the 'moral' deficiency of the individual in the deserving/undeserving discourse. While it is true that the Great Recession gave new momentum, in Britain and elsewhere in the world, to the anti-scrounger rhetoric, the post-recession context has opened up new landscapes. The emergence of the refugee crisis in Europe is only one element of a new social crisis that brings about new dichotomies in our society and inevitably also affects the formulation of dominant views about deservedness in the welfare state.

Notes

1 YouGov/TUC Survey Results, Fieldwork, 12–12 December 2012, available at www.tuc.org.uk/sites/default/files/Welfarepoll_summaryresults.pdf.
2 It should be noted that during 2007 and 2009 the answer 'because they are not doing enough' was substituted with 'because they live beyond their means'. As both answers refer to the imputed individual behaviour of the person and do not alter the general result of the analysis, they are left unchanged in our discussion.
3 Declaration of Chancellor George Osborne at Prime Minister's questions, *The Guardian*, 17 June 2015: 'We can either continue on a completely unsustainable path or we can continue reforming welfare so that work pays and we give a fair deal to those on welfare and indeed a fair deal to the people, the taxpayers of this country, who pay for it.'
4 Word cloud is a technique used to represent in a visual manner the frequency of occurrence of terms in a given text or discussion.

Part III
Insiders and outsiders

7 Geographies of solidarity

Immigrants and the city

We open the third and last section of this volume with a chapter on the spatial dimension of inclusion and solidarity. In the first part of the book the notion of solidarity has been predominantly discussed from the standpoint of the *moral* background of a given society in its relationships with the 'deserving' ones, while Part II was devoted to the analysis of the *social* representations of deservedness and undeservedness and their how these ideas are understood among the general public. This chapter looks at the spatial dimension of both solidarity and inclusion based on the idea that social separations are not centred on moral and social boundaries alone: geographical divisions can also have a powerful role in creating or re-enforcing isolation and exclusion, a process which sociologist Loïc Wacquant (1993; 1996) has termed 'territorial stigmatisation'. This is not only a topical issue in the scientific and political arena but also a significant element in our overall discussion of the social and moral backgrounds of solidarity and in our analysis of the possible differences between the Anglo-Saxon and Mediterranean models. Few would say that solidarity is not strictly linked to the spatial dimension, a relationship that becomes immediately evident as soon as we accept Ruth Lupton's notion of *neighbourhoods* as not 'just physical spaces but as complex and overlapping webs of social relationships' (2003: 16). Having said this, our intention in the present chapter is to complement the analysis made so far in the book with a discussion of the different geographies of solidarities in an Italian and a British city, Naples and London respectively. This comparison will be made from a specific point of view, that of young immigrants and their relationship with the urban context.

One of the most fascinating themes in urban studies is the incredible variety of potential diverse patterns of interaction between immigrants and urban spaces in different geographical contexts. How immigrants settle in host cities, experience their life in the neighbourhood, interact with the local community and even change the environment they live in are all recurring subjects of investigation in sociology, anthropology, geography, demography, economics, urban, cultural and migration studies, just to mention a few. Moreover, given their inherent dynamic features, these patterns are perennial themes for discussion and an inexhaustible territory for research.

It is significant however that the bulk of research on immigrant communities in urban contexts has long privileged spatial *marginality* as a field of analysis. The vast literature on the modern *ghetto* is the most representative of this stream of research.[1] We owe a debt to the Chicago School of sociology and to the work of Robert E. Park, and Louis Wirth in particular, not only for the first comprehensive empirical analysis of the ghetto in America but also for the first attempt at describing it in sociological terms. Wirth's enquiry into the Chicago ghetto (1927, 1928) has been criticised for its deterministic approach – the idea that immigrant culture will reproduce itself in these settlements; but their work remains fundamental even today, most importantly because they identified spatial marginality as an important common feature of Jewish ghettos and their equivalents of the time (such as the Italian *Little Sicily* or Chinese *Chinatowns*). Some of Wirth's critics have firmly opposed the idea that these spatial formations all emerged as poles of attraction for migrant communities with a similar 'economic status and cultural tradition' (1928: 283), and in fact have made a clear distinction between the ghetto and the *ethnic enclave*, the latter notable for a much more 'diluted' concentration of ethnicity than the 'black ghetto' (Peach, 2005: 38).[2]

Regardless of these critiques, the Chicago School of sociology's research into the life of European and African-American communities in urban settlements can be said to represent a fundamental step for the sociological understanding of the relationships between social and spatial isolation. It evidenced, among other things, a parallel between patterns of marginality or 'social distance' among minorities and their residential concentration in specific urban areas of American cities (Wirth, 1928; Burgess, 1928) which remained a central analytical key even for the description of new spatial configurations in the post-Fordist city.[3]

Over the second part of the twentieth century, a number of economic and urban dynamics came to transform the centre/periphery relationships in major cities. Especially, but not exclusively, in North American metropolitan areas the urbanisation process reached saturation point during the 1970s, making city centres less attractive for the middle class. Urban and industrial restructuring, together with the movement of the upper and middle class towards the suburbs altered the historical role of urban centres as the economic and social core of the city. With residential differentiation by *neighbourhood* being substituted by separation in different metropolitan macro-areas, the social distance of the urban poor of the city from the wealthy part of society became increasingly more pronounced. These dynamics made the role of urban spatial separation even more evident. W. J. Wilson's studies on urban poverty, for example (1978, 1987, 1988), showed that a 'concentration effect' occurs not only within immigrant ghettos but also for all inhabitants of poor neighbourhoods of the inner city, i.e. the 'underclass' and in particular its African-descended component.

Wilson's ideas on economic class-based separation complementing racial–ethnic segregation shed new light on the significance of the urban 'ghetto' at the end of the century:[4] a deprived urban area with a high concentration of poor and unemployed people; a distinctive 'social milieu' characterised by social disadvantage, isolation and the exclusion of its inhabitants from job networks, social capital and inclusion opportunities that are generally found in other non-deprived areas. Wilson (1987: 56) suggested that the historical departure of wealthy working-class families from inner-city areas for suburbia deprived neighbourhood communities of a fundamental 'social buffer' that would effectively reduce the impact of joblessness and social exclusion. Studies by Wilson and others showed, as a consequence, that the post-Fordist ghetto cannot be understood simply as a space of religious, ethnic and racial separation but must also, and increasingly so in the *hyper-ghetto*, be viewed as a territorial enclave based on economic segregation exacerbated by 'mutually reinforcing' transformations (Wacquant and Wilson, 1993: 28).

This stream of the literature had a prominent role in paving the way for a more profound analysis of the new 'outcast' ghetto (Marcuse, 1996; Marcuse, 1997) and urban spatial marginality in general as a distinctive phenomenon of contemporary cities both in the US and in Europe. Today scholars predominantly distinguish between at least two main *regimes* of advanced marginality in Western cities, with the US and the British model typified by persisting 'rigid spatial and social separation' (Wacquant, 1998: 1640) and even hyper-segregation along racial, ethnic and class boundaries (Massey and Denton, 1989; Wilkes and Iceland, 2004; Burgess et al., 2005; Morawska, 2009; Massey and Tannen, 2015).[5] The European pattern has displayed a less pronounced model of residential segregation, partly as an effect of the historical role played by the welfare state and municipal governance in attenuating the detrimental effects of modernism (Mingione, 1996; Wacquant, 1996; Bagnasco and Le Galés, 2000; Häussermann, 2005; Häussermann and Haila, 2005). However, when the sole category of immigrants and ethnic minorities is considered, spatial concentration and segregation is found also within European cities, albeit at a much lower degree than in the US and in spite of great variation at country and city levels (Musterd, 2005; Van Kempen, 2005; Östh et al., 2015). One fitting example of these dynamics regards the centre/periphery polarisation, whose relationship is apparently 'reversed' (Harvey, 1996: 38) in some European cities as opposed to the US model, with suburban realities (such as the French *banlieues*) revealing much profound 'suffering', isolation and segregation among immigrants and minorities than the gentrified inner city (Wacquant, 2007).

Whatever their specific configuration, spatial inequality and urban segregation can be said to stand as central elements in the analysis of immigrant isolation and vulnerability in contemporary cities. However, and despite an incredible amount of research devoted to these issues, almost 30 years after the appearance of Wilson's work on the concentration effects in poor neighbourhoods our understanding of spatial inequality and its dynamics is still incomplete, and even the notion of a (detrimental) neighbourhood effect is far from being universally agreed on in the literature. A number of scholars, for example, have contended that one cannot properly talk of neighbourhood effects if the concentration of poor and unemployed people in socially isolated areas is the mere result of a *self-selection* process led by housing markets and income-based residential choices (Cheshire, 2007). All in all, this part of the scholarship insists, urban social segregation is the 'reflection' of economic inequality rather than its cause.

While it is evident that concentration effects are less detrimental to working- and middle-class families who voluntarily move to a certain residential area, the same argument is much more debatable when one considers that most long-term unemployed and poor families may not have the same *freedom of choice* when deciding where to live (Sen, 1992).

It is true, as a rich body of literature has shown over the years, that residential segregation is often derived from a clear preference of immigrants and minorities for neighbourhoods that already display a strong ethnic concentration (Marcuse, 2005; Van der Laan Bouma-Doff, 2007; Van Ham and Manley, 2015). However, two aspects should be taken into consideration. Firstly, immigrants, and low-income newcomers in particular, constitute a specific category of vulnerable population, thus particularly exposed to the effects of *economically forced residential segregation* in host societies. Secondly, the overall preference of natives for residing in neighbourhoods with no ethnic minority has also led to the intensification of the concentration effect (Semyonov and Herring, 2007).

Therefore, and regardless of whether ethnic and social concentration is caused by voluntary or involuntary clustering processes, the *objective* impact of spatial isolation on social inequalities and poverty remains undeniable when we look at its effects in terms of health (McLaughlin et al., 2007; Ludwig et al., 2012), education (Lipman, 2011), the labour market (Bayer et al., 2004) and social inclusion in general.

Research conducted on the latter theme has convincingly illustrated the extent to which spatial isolation may negatively affect access to informal job-search channels and to important social capital networks. The recent resurgence of 'social mix' experimental plans used in European and US cities to artificially 'rebalance' the socio-economic composition of neighbourhoods is indicative of the growing attention devoted (both in academic and political arenas) to understanding and combating the persistent negative effects of spatial inequalities on individual opportunities.[6] In this regard, however, an increasing body of critical scholarship has called into question the real impact of social mix strategies by empirically demonstrating that these policies do not necessarily eliminate the causes of poverty and social exclusion, mainly because there is little interaction between inhabitants of artificially mixed communities (Ostendorf et al., 2001; Gilbert, 2009; Manley et al., 2012). These results point to the fact that not only does physical proximity have a central role in augmenting social inclusion; so too do social networks, and especially in the case of immigrants. They also call for a more comprehensive understanding of the links between urban spatial inclusion and social networks of migrant people, something which we intend to address in the remaining sections of this chapter by examining the spatial inclusion of immigrants in two European cities: Naples and London.

Spatial inclusion and solidarity: urban lives of young low-income immigrants in Naples and London

Objectives of the study and method

The main purpose of the analysis presented here is to expand our knowledge of the dynamics regulating urban inclusion and exclusion of immigrants by looking at one of the most recurring research themes in urban studies – the spatial inclusion of migrants – together with another dimension which is much less explored: that of solidarity patterns of immigrants both with their own community and with the host population. It is worth clarifying that the purpose in this chapter is not to provide an account of the spatial dimension of poverty or inequality among the migrant poor, or to investigate their solidarity networks within the immigrant community. There is already a great deal of past and contemporary literature addressing the theme of solidarity *among* immigrants and *towards* them. To a far lesser extent have scholars dealt with immigrants' configurations of solidarity *with* host societies and possibly with other immigrant communities settled in their geographical area. The objective of this study, therefore, is to explore the 'neighbourhood experience' of migrant residents as a whole.

The starting point of the research relies on two simple propositions: firstly, solidarity is at the same time a key component in the lives of those who experience temporary or permanent vulnerability (one could even say a means of 'survival') and a major dimension in social cohesion, inclusion and integration. As such, it is a vital element in the lives of immigrants. To begin with, and given the overall aims of this volume, an analysis of spatial inclusion and solidarity patterns of immigrants in Naples and London provides further elements for the discussion and comparison of the solidarity models of Italy and Great Britain. Secondly, our comparison will contribute further to the description of these two cities and their apparent differences in terms of urban and social configuration. More specifically, the focus on these two cases can shed new light on the existence of different regimes of urban marginality in the European and Anglo-Saxon worlds. We will test in particular the common assumption that urban ghettos have not developed in European cities partly as an effect of the peculiar model of social 'aggregation' of Continental Europe (Wacquant, 1996) and that of London as an exception to this model, with residential segregation of immigrants being a distinctive characteristic of its spatial configuration.

In order to do so, the study centres on three predominant questions. Firstly, how *spatially integrated* are immigrants, not only from the point of view of their residence but also in terms of occupation and social activities? In other words, how do immigrants experience the urban space they live in? Secondly, does solidarity have a role in the inclusion and integration of immigrants into that urban space? Thirdly, what are the main differences between London and Naples in terms of neighbourhood cohesion and local forms of interaction of immigrants with their community and the host society?

The study presented in the following sections is based on original material from interviews conducted in the cities of London and Naples during 2015 and 2016. At the time of the interviews a purposive (i.e. non-representative) sample of low-income working immigrants aged 18–36 residing and working in the areas of Naples and London was identified through online advertisements and word of mouth within the interviewees' networks.[7] A total of 40 respondents (17 women and 23 men) were recruited, of 25 different nationalities. Data was collected during face-to-face interviews conducted via a semi-structured questionnaire comprising structured questions on the interviewees' socio-demographic characteristics, home and work addresses and semi-structured questions addressing their spatial inclusion, solidarity and neighbourhood relationships.

Neighbourhoods of London and Naples

At least since the appearance of Charles Booth's inquiry into 'The Life and Labour of the People in London' (first published 1889), social and economic conditions in the British capital have been mapped, represented and studied with incessant interest. Among other things, Booth's study famously provided a geographical representation of urban configurations of poverty, and his maps are still used today to observe and compare the persisting spatial patterns of marginality in London (see for example Orford et al., 2002). With respect to these configurations, the relevant literature identifies two main elements that can be said to be characteristic of the London area. The first is the profound impact of the immigrant population on the urban development of the city, and in particular on the *spatial concentration* of ethnic populations in specific parts of the metropolitan space. While empirical research on different areas of London generally confirms that ethnic segregation is a persistent, distinctive feature of the city, most of the scholarship recognises that the residential concentration of ethnic minorities in Britain cannot be equated with the urban configurations of North American cities (i.e. the urban ghetto) both in terms of its *extent* (ethnic concentration levels are much lower in London than in American cities) and for its *impact* on marginalisation processes (residential segregation in London does not seem to exacerbate social exclusion and discrimination as is the case in the hyper-ghetto) (Peach, 1996; Peach, 2005; Peach, 2009; Johnston et al., 2002a; Johnston et al., 2002b; Johnston et al., 2007; Brimicombe, 2007; Finney and Simpson, 2009).

A second recurring element in the description of London concerns the *gentrification* process and its changing patterns over the years. Broadly defined as 'the transformation of a working class or a vacant area of the central city into middle-class residential and/or commercial use' (Lees et al., 2008: xv), the notion of gentrification was first used in the literature precisely to designate a phenomenon distinctive to the London area (Glass, 1964 [2010]), only to become a recurring theme of urban studies throughout the world since the mid-1960s (Palen and London, 1984; Smith, 1996; Lees, 2000; Atkinson and Bridge, 2005). The return of the middle class from suburban areas to the inner city remains a topical issue to keep in mind as far as London is concerned, and in particular for its effects on the reconfiguration of spatial inequality in the city: the repopulation of inner cities comes in conjunction with the expulsion/replacement of those inhabitants who got 'priced out' of the local housing market (Hamnett, 2003: 163) and their movement to more affordable neighbourhoods or parts of neighbourhoods. It has been noted that such a process in some cases augments both social segregation and social distance at the 'micro' level between wealthy gentrifiers and other settlers (Atkinson, 2000a; Atkinson, 2000b; Butler, 2003; Butler and Lees, 2006; Higgins et al., 2014). Two apparently opposing forces – residential socio-ethnic segregation and the dispersion of middle-class families across affordable areas of the city – are, however, only two aspects of the complex constellation of urban development dynamics in London[8] that amplify a process anticipated by Ruth Glass in the 1960s: the transformation of the British capital into a space dominated by the 'survival of the [financial] fittest' for its inhabitants (1964: 23).[9]

The city of Naples could not appear more different from London, at least at first sight. At a general level, there is a profound difference between these cities in terms of geographical extension, population size, economy and demography which makes the two cases apparently 'incomparable'. Furthermore, it is evident that Naples lacks both the fluidity and the pace of the urban transformations which are characteristic of the British capital while being at the same time the quintessence of fluidity itself: a 'multiform' urban space, an 'extraordinary kaleidoscope' resulting from the sum of 'different cities' (Becchi, 1989: 145–147) wherein the urban landscape is strongly fragmented by the different functions and historical identities of each neighbourhood (Laino, 2014).

But above all, and of major interest to our discussion, there is the differing scale of the immigrant populations living in the two cities, with Naples displaying a much lower share of foreign-born people relative to the overall population (4–5 per cent in 2015)[10] than inner London (39 per cent in 2014),[11] something which has long led many commentators to consider Naples exclusively in terms of a 'transit destination' for immigrants (for a discussion and recent trends see De Filippo et al., 2010; Harney, 2011). There is no doubt that the traditional absence of ethnic enclaves in Naples (Morlicchio and Pugliese, 2006) has been increasingly altered by new forms of spatial distribution of the immigrant population across different neighbourhoods. In some cases, new immigration flows have produced both a significant concentration of certain ethnic groups in specific areas of the inner city and the appropriation of public spaces for recreational and work activities (Dines, 2012; Russo Krauss, 2014).

Another distinctive element which is generally mentioned when the city of Naples is considered is the massive role played by local practices of mutual help and solidarity at the neighbourhood level. Ethnographic accounts of life in Naples' districts, or *rioni*, have long stressed how solidarity among neighbours is not only a moral duty but also and predominantly a strategic means of local *negotiation* through which resources and power are distributed, conceded or denied to family, friends and neighbours (Pardo, 1996: 95).

In spite of the above-mentioned differences, recent research shows that in some parts of London the *neighbourhood* remains an important 'resource in terms of reciprocity' (Beaumont, 2006: 149) both for native households and migrant individuals living far from home. In particular, the work of Datta on London immigrants and their spatial practices of interaction with the 'local' and the 'translocal' provides a new, fitting conceptualisation of the neighbourhood, seen as 'a day-to-day mundane negotiation of the particular localized opportunities that can evoke notions of home and belonging' (2011: 75). Such an emphasis on the role of neighbourhoods as instruments of *survival* and *negotiation* – rather than mere places of integration or assimilation – is something which encourages further exploration of the possible similarities between Naples and the British metropolis.

Casa e puteca: spatial inclusion of young immigrants in everyday life

> I moved from Caserta to Naples because I was feeling too lonely. In Caserta I had a good full-time job but the loneliness was too great so I decided to go to Naples where all my community is.
>
> (Mudi, aged 32, arrived in 2006)

A common assumption made about the ethnic segregation of immigrants across the urban space is that it is best measured by their *residential concentration* by ethnicity or nationality. Only to a lesser degree has the spatial dimension of the *work* and *social life* of immigrants been taken into account in order to discuss their spatial inclusion in the host society (Ellis et al., 2004; Wissink et al., 2016). Bearing in mind that the object of this study is *young* working immigrants, their spatial experience of the city for working activities and social purposes alike should be considered of major importance together with their residential distribution. The first set of questions asked our respondents specifically about their relationship with the urban context. We asked all respondents to provide their last two home addresses and to explain the reason for deciding to live in their present neighbourhood. We also asked them to indicate their current work address and to indicate some of the places they most frequently go to with friends or family for recreational purposes. In order to obtain a general overview of how our respondents experience the urban space, face-to-face interview analysis is combined with observation of the spatial distribution of their residence, work address and social activities. Most of those interviewed provided names of neighbourhood associations, restaurants, clubs or bars and addresses of friends, but many also indicated public spaces such as squares, parks and markets as the most visited places to gather and meet friends or family.

The maps provided here synthesise the urban experience of our respondents as obtained from the conversion of home/work addresses and the most frequent spaces of aggregation into geographic coordinates. They obviously do not intend to provide a representative illustration of residential or work distribution. Rather, they should be read as complementary visual tools with which to discuss results from our interviews. An interesting general result from this first set of questions is that none of the respondents felt that he or she was constrained by economic or social reasons to live at the present address. All of the interviewees showed a strong awareness concerning their decision, and most of them said that they were satisfied with their current place of residence. In terms of residential distribution, as expected and consistent with empirical findings from the most recent literature, the majority of the immigrants interviewed in Naples live and work in the inner city, as Figure 7.1 illustrates. Also, most of the respondents' social lives are concentrated around the historic centre of the city, and predominantly around its eastern side. If we look away from the Naples municipality and focus on the overall spatial distribution of immigrants across the greater Naples area, their spatial concentration in the centre appears much more visible, with only one immigrant worker commuting outside the city's municipal area (Figure 7.2).

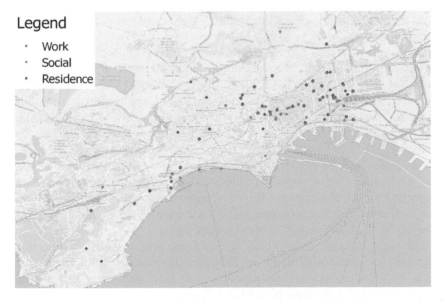

Figure 7.1 Spatial distribution of residence, work and social spaces for a sample of immigrants in the City of Naples, 2015–2016
Source: Author's elaboration of data obtained with Quantum GIS, Open Source Geospatial Foundation Project. http://qgis.osgeo.org.

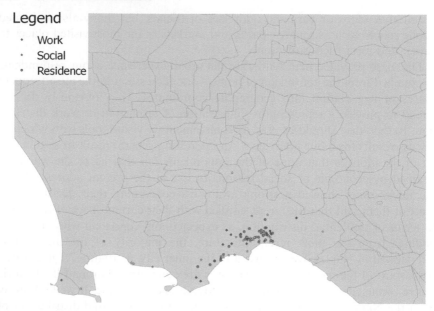

Figure 7.2 Spatial distribution of residence, work and social spaces for a sample of
immigrants in the Province of Naples, 2015–2016
Source: Author's elaboration of data obtained with Quantum GIS, Open Source
Geospatial Foundation Project. http://qgis.osgeo.org.

As for residential choices and their motives, although most of our interviewees
mention the convenient location of their present address in terms of distance
from work and access to public transport, by and large all of those interviewed in Naples identify the presence of family, community or friends from
home[12] as the main reason for going to live in the area. However, a distinction
can be made based on nationality. Arabic-speaking immigrants from different
countries of the Maghreb region, for example, seem to be strongly 'attached'
to the area surrounding the central railway station (Piazza Garibaldi) for their
residence. While this may be unsurprising given the strong presence of immigrants in this part of the city, it is the growing role of this area as a 'multi-
functional space' for foreigners (Dines, 2003: 177) that constitutes the most
important factor of attraction for our respondents – the daily *social* life of
Piazza Garibaldi where one can meet a member of the community at 'any
time of the day', as one of the interviewees said.

The short distance from work, at the same time, appears of major significance for immigrants living in the area. For many employed in shops,
stalls, fast-food kiosks or restaurants in the Garibaldi area, living nearby
is seen as part of a strategic plan to save both resources and commuting time,
something which one respondent poignantly described as *fare casa e puteca*.[13]
For others however, living in the proximity of the 'social' centre of the city is
not seen as a priority. This is especially true for Asian immigrants (most

notably from Sri Lanka and India), who undoubtedly tend to be more concentrated in terms of residence and rarely mention proximity to spaces of social aggregation as a reason to live in a specific area. As is the case for Mudi, a part-time care-giver whose story is mentioned at the beginning of this section, *loneliness* can be a sufficient reason for moving away from a settlement and reuniting with the native community regardless of economic and working insecurity.

On the other hand, however, Asian immigrants seem to use a greater part of the urban space for their social and recreational activities as compared to immigrants from Arabic countries. The use of parks and big open spaces by young members of the Sri Lankan and Indian community for a game of cricket or a picnic has become a regular phenomenon which attests to the increasing appropriation of different parts of the city by one part of the immigrant population.

These patterns are not so evident in the case of London, where rationales for residential choices are really mixed. In terms of spatial distribution, two main aspects are immediately notable from Figure 7.3: firstly, it is evident that immigrants in the London area rarely live in the city centre (indicated by the large star in the illustration). Although many of them work in London city, the majority of our respondents' residences are located in peripheral neighbourhoods of London or in Greater London.

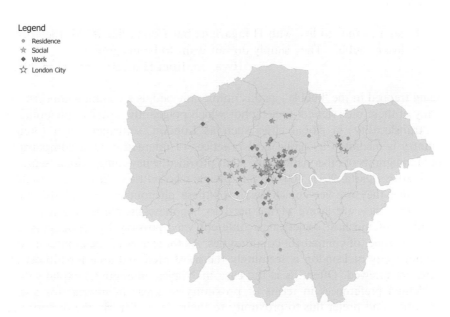

Figure 7.3 Spatial distribution of residence, work and social spaces for a sample of immigrants in the Greater London area, 2015–2016
Source: Author's elaboration of data obtained with Quantum GIS, Open Source Geospatial Foundation Project. http://qgis.osgeo.org.

In terms of residential choices, results are very mixed. Some of our respondents confirmed that the presence of family or members of their community in the same neighbourhood (or even in the same flat) was a main factor driving the decision. However, for many (especially those who live with a partner or children) there is the explicit intention of finding a quiet, safe or green neighbourhood in London in which to live and to improve their quality of life by moving away from an isolated or degraded area. It is also frequently the case that the decision was affected by the emergence of a good opportunity to rent a flat or room left by compatriots, something which in many cases led them to share accommodation with other immigrants of the same nationality despite not intending to do so. An interesting finding from the analysis of London immigrants' rationales for residential choices concerns the frequent decision *not* to live in neighbourhoods where the presence of compatriots is very strong. This is a common result found during many of the interviews. When asked to expand on the reasons for living in a particular neighbourhood, many (especially the youngest in the London sample) explicitly referred to a strong personal desire not to reside in close proximity to fellow nationals in order to improve one's language skills and facilitate integration with British people and immigrants of other nationalities. This belief, for many young immigrants interviewed, is mainly derived from the experience of compatriots who failed in their migratory project in terms of social integration:

> I had a chance to live with Hungarians but I don't like it. All they do is to live in bubble. They simply do not want to be integrated.
>
> (Eva, 25, from Hungary, arrived in 2013)

Being trapped in the 'bubble', as this immigrant said, is a common concern for many of those interviewed, a metaphor which poignantly describes phenomena of 'translocality' in global cities such as London: settlement in a foreign country is mediated by daily local practices of interaction with compatriots and immigrants of other nationalities that provide the newcomer with a 'sense of familiarity' (Datta, 2011: 100). Young people who refuse to 'live in the bubble' show that they are very much aware of these phenomena and, at the same time, that they are aware of the need to negotiate their integration as full members of the host society in a different way, possibly by renouncing the 'comfort zone' of compatriot communities. As for spaces of social interaction, the inner city of London is seemingly the most preferred area for almost all those interviewed. Often, as is the case in Naples, immigrants explain their residential preferences in terms of proximity to areas of interest for social recreation and prefer this to proximity to their place of work, the opposite of many cases in London. However, there is a striking difference between the two cases as immigrants in London indicate their preferred areas for social recreation based on the concentration of entertainment opportunities (art exhibitions, music performances, pubs, fitness classes and so on), while

Neapolitan immigrants more frequently refer to the proximity of areas where compatriots tend to gather. Another significant difference worth noting between the two cases is the presence of relatives or members of their community in the neighbourhood of residence: in Naples it is more common to have a family or community member in the neighbourhood than in London, but among London immigrants who say so, it is much more frequent than in Naples for the interviewee to share a flat or a room with one or more of them.

'With a little help' from the community: solidarity and rainy days

One of the central points in our study regarded the role of solidarity for young immigrants living far from home. All of our respondents were asked whether they had experienced any financial difficulty over the past two years and who, if anyone, had helped them. We were particularly interested in two aspects: the role of institutional forms of social support (i.e. welfare benefits) and the use of local and community networks of solidarity. An initial common finding for all respondents in both Naples and London is the rare resort to institutional forms of support. Only in three cases did we find someone who received unemployment support (one in Naples and two in London), albeit for a very short amount of time. Another two persons said that they received family or children transfers. With the exception of these respondents, most of those interviewed did experience economic problems for different reasons (temporary unemployment, health problems, low income and unexpected costs are the most common causes mentioned) but never applied for benefits. Most of these believed that they would be ineligible or feared that applying for benefits would eventually worsen their situation.

> I never considered claiming social benefits even when I had economic difficulties. It is a trap, [it is] too comfortable, you do not aspire to do more and got stuck.
>
> (Catia, 30, from Portugal, arrived in 2011)

Claiming benefits is generally regarded as a failure, especially for the youngest among our interviewees, who fiercely often admit that they managed to resolve their problems 'on their own', by doing extra work or by cutting down on expenses. However, the most frequent method for coping with economic problems for immigrants in both Naples and London is help from family and close friends, most often in the form of a personal loan from parents, relatives or members of the native community. This is especially relevant in the Neapolitan case where, besides parents, it is the *local linguistic-ethnic community* that young members turn to most often when in need, regardless of their level of interaction with Italians and other communities. For many of those interviewed, helping and receiving help from one's own native community is something one can rely on. Mourad, a

38-year-old Algerian who settled in Naples in 1999, explains that economic support (but also social and psychological assistance) is something that cannot be refused to members of the community who are experiencing problems in a foreign country:

> Help among compatriots is a duty. If an old person gets sick or a member of the community is hospitalised, you must go and visit, bring food, offer your assistance.

Being compatriots is described by Mourad as a sufficient reason for feeling obliged to help, even years after first arriving in a country. On one occasion, he remembers paying for a hotel room for a woman and her children (who he had never met before) arriving in Naples from the Maghreb region because they needed a place to stay for a couple of days. This and many other stories collected in Naples indicate that immigrants in this city base much of their solidarity and survival strategies on the social support of the community, and not only in financial terms. Clothes and food exchange, material help (like baby-sitting or assistance to the elderly), offering a room and collecting money for funerals or health emergencies are among the most commonly mentioned practices of solidarity within the immigrant communities we met. We also investigated solidarity from and with the Italian community. According to our interviewees, this is most often provided by Neapolitans in the form of general 'logistic' support (help to find a room or a job, information and assistance with bureaucracy). Financial help from Italians is also mentioned (one young person said that he received financial help to buy a scooter; another received some cash to pay for a rent deposit for a flat), but this appears to be something which immigrants rarely resort to.

Finally, most of the respondents said that they had never had the chance to help a Neapolitan. A minor but interesting exception to this trend is provided by Muslim immigrants who practice *zakat* (a fixed sum of alms paid out of personal revenues and wealth) and *sadaquat* (voluntary almsgiving). One of the five pillars of Islam, almsgiving in general is considered an important duty, and all of the Muslims we interviewed said that they do *zakat* in Naples by devolving their voluntary almsgiving according to a 'proximity' rule. Regardless of nationality, they accord a sum of money or food to those members of society (including Neapolitans and members of other nationalities who live in Naples) who are closest to them and in need.[14]

The London case reveals much laxer ties in the native community. Here young people tend to ask for help when necessary in order to go on with their migratory project, and only turn to those they feel they can really trust. Much more frequently than their Neapolitan counterparts, immigrants in London report that they only ask their family or closest friends for help regardless of their nationality. The main reason for that, in the words of many interviewees, is the worry about *social expectations* on the part of those who helped, as a Nigerian woman told us:

[In London] everything is based on the survival of the fittest, reciprocity is the rule, you help others but only if you are really close and can expect to receive help when you are in need, it is never for free.

(Christine, 29, arrived in London 2014)

London immigrants show that they are fully aware of rules regulating help as a form of 'gift', which is given spontaneously but based on the tacit assumption that reciprocity will follow (Mauss, 1954). It is unsurprising then that many among the immigrants we interviewed consider very carefully who can be helped and who can help in return, a sort of survival strategy for young people living in a foreign country.

I just don't want to put myself in a vulnerable position. If I leave [compatriots] enter my life, I become vulnerable to their constant requests for help and I cannot afford this.

(Michalina, 22, from Poland, arrived in London 2012)

This, however, is not to say that networks of solidarity and support do not exist among London immigrants. On the contrary, besides help from close family, our interviewees frequently report stories of transnational networks of mutual help and assistance. Almost all of those interviewed have hosted an acquaintance (either a fellow national or those of other nationalities) in need of a room at least once since their arrival, and many have lent money to one or more friends. Unlike Naples, it is not common for immigrants in London to give each other material help. Networks of solidarity entailing the exchange of clothes or food and the collection of money are found, but they predominantly occur through formal channels, e.g. local charitable associations and community centres. These forms of support, however, seem to be the prerogative of long-term settlers or of the oldest in the sample. At the same time, helping others is very common among those we interviewed. It is common to be involved in a volunteering activity (charities, homelessness shelters, food banks, independent trade unions and cat sanctuaries are mentioned), but it is rarer in comparison with Naples for London immigrants to provide material help with children or the elderly from the community.

Do you know your neighbours?

Our overall expectation with regard to neighbourhood relations was mixed. On the one hand, if it is true that residential segregation by nationality is pronounced as a phenomenon in London, we should expect social and community relations to be strong at the neighbourhood level. On the other hand, however, this would require exclusive interaction with members of the same nationality rather than interaction with locals. For the Neapolitan case, it was predicted that interaction with neighbours would be stronger than in the London case, both because the residential concentration of immigrants is lower and due to the distinctive forms of social interaction there. A single, open question dominated the last part of our interview: *Do you know your neighbours?* A first piece of information resulting from the interviews should be mentioned, and concerns the presence of two very diverse situations in Naples and London: most London immigrants reported that they never had the chance to meet the neighbours, either because the person next door has just moved in or because they have just arrived themselves. With a few exceptions, it is also very rare for them to know someone in the building or in the immediate area in general. Furthermore, London immigrants tend to attribute the lack of social interaction with neighbours to the fact that, for the majority, these people are immigrant families and they have little interest in befriending them. Conversely, most immigrants living in Naples know their neighbours regardless of the duration of their stay at the present address and of the building's composition in terms of nationality.

Having said this, we can analyse our findings from the interviews by referring to two main themes. The first and more important is, once again, the different practices of negotiation in Naples and London. Some of the immigrant workers in London say they know who the neighbours are: they can recognise them and occasionally greet them, but overall it is very rare for the interaction to go further than that. Interestingly, for some of the respondents this situation is normal. They have never contemplated the possibility of visiting a neighbour or asking for some form of help, and anyway it is often felt that they would have no time to build such relationships. For others, on the other hand, the lack of social interaction with those living in the same building is felt as the 'sad' consequence of settling in a big city. Young people from Southern European countries in particular reported they have sometimes attempted to befriend a neighbour but they lost interest after their initial effort had not been reciprocated. On the other hand, immigrants in the Neapolitan context seem more involved in social interactions at the neighbourhood level, be it in the form of social interaction, friendship or social support among neighbours. Four reactions from our interviews can help illustrate the different patterns found in Naples and London:

We [me and my neighbours] have a normal relationship, sometimes we watch the football match together, sometimes we drink coffee, we chat, it is the kind of normal relationship you have with neighbours.

(Nadim, 28, from Algeria, arrived in Naples in 2012)

I know the lady next door, of course. We talk every day; we take coffee, if there is a problem in the building we discuss what is going on and things like that.

(Fatima, 34, from Ivory Coast, arrived in Naples in 2000)

Back in the days I had an English neighbour that I knew personally; we would occasionally have a talk. Then he moved away and immigrants came in but I never had the opportunity to know them.

(Amesh, 29, from India, arrived in London in 2005)

We used to meet an old couple in the building, spending Christmas time and the holidays together every year with my children. Now we do not meet anymore, they live in another neighbourhood and there is no time to visit.

(Kemelia, 36, from Bulgaria, arrived in London in 2007)

The voices of Fatima and Nadim can be viewed as representative of most of those interviewed in Naples. Regular relationships with neighbours in their words are felt as natural and sometimes even unavoidable when something occurs in the building. This applies both to immigrants living alone and to those who have an Italian partner who was born and raised in the area. Yet these immigrants never consider neighbourhood relations in terms of a social obligation. Inviting someone over for a coffee in Naples is a regular daily practice, but also a gesture full of social meaning, a practice that many of the interviewees reveal they have become accustomed to.

In London, conversely, a self-defence approach of immigrants is the predominating tendency. There is always a 'missed' opportunity or lack of time to get to know one's neighbours; but at the same time it is not uncommon for many of the respondents to express a feeling of indifference or discomfort when talking about neighbourhood relations. An aspect that can be considered of some importance, however, is the fact that many immigrants in London share their apartment with others. It is possible that the 'roommate' community in this situation can perform the functions of the local community, acting as a 'micro-neighbourhood' where networks of exchange, solidarity and support are created.

This point leads us to the second and final element emerging from the interviews, which is the immigrants' relationships with the neighbourhood as a space. Although many of the respondents in London stated that they chose their present address because it is located in a nice area, only few can be said to experience the neighbourhood in a proper way. It is very common for young immigrants to leave for work in the morning only to come back home late in the evening, possibly following social encounters with friends in the immediate proximity of work or in central areas of London. Examining responses in the London case, we are tempted to say that those interviewed often experience their neighbourhood as 'phantom inhabitants'. Since there is no real record of social interaction with the local community or its main activities, these neighbourhoods are predominantly used by young immigrants (especially those without children) as 'bedroom communities'. What strikes one most about this finding, however, is not only that suburban areas of London are subject to this phenomenon; so too are central boroughs such as Camden or Fulham.

If we compare this result with Naples, the situation could not seem more different. Of course, working immigrants in the Naples area also have only a few hours per day to spend in their neighbourhood. Nevertheless, as already mentioned, the local neighbourhood is often not only a place of residence but also a meeting place where, according to immigrants, they frequently go at the end of the day to buy food, meet friends or just have a walk with their partner.

Naples and London: between survival and negotiation

In one of the first studies on the topic, Robert A. Woods wrote that 'the neighbourhood is large enough to include in essence all the problems of the city, the state, and the nation' (1914: 578). In a similar way, we can conclude this chapter by considering the discussion of the neighbourhood as illustrative of the whole study. Life in the neighbourhood is not incomparable in the two cities. However, the different patterns of interaction of immigrants with their local communities remain an interesting sociological result. Do our findings confirm our predictions on the spatial relations of immigrants with the city? To some extent, they do not. Contrary to predictions and to general assumptions that see London's immigrants living in strong geographical proximity, the respondents' answers tell us a different story. Young people try to escape the 'bubble' of their compatriots' community, and their relationships with the local context are by and large dominated by sentiments of indifference. Conversely, the Neapolitan context in some way confirms our expectations, especially in terms of solidarity networks among immigrants. However, this finding seems to be strongly associated with the increasing residential concentration of immigrants in certain areas of the historic centre for different reasons.

In terms of the social and spatial distance of immigrants from the local communities of Naples and London, two central aspects should be mentioned. Firstly, there is in Naples a strong preference among immigrants for interactions with those of the same nationality for social and recreation purposes, something which appears less evident in the London context, where young immigrants frequently interact with people from many different nationalities. Secondly and despite this, feelings of loneliness are much more frequent in the London sample. A common element in most of our conversations with immigrants is the incapacity to establish in the host city 'a true friendship like those I used to have back home', something which many young people in London said they try to confront by attending volunteering activities, meet-ups and fitness classes. Conversely, while this theme never emerged in our discussion with immigrants in Naples, it is undeniable that their social and spatial inclusion is still achieved only in part. Young immigrants in Naples rarely mention social activities like going to the cinema, attending a music event or partaking in a sports class as something they do on a regular or even an occasional basis. Furthermore, their 'experience' of the urban context, unlike their London counterparts, is still strongly linked to the place of residence or areas of social aggregation for immigrants.

We can conclude our chapter by noting that in one aspect London and Naples can be said to be similar – that is in terms of their role as spaces of constant negotiation and efforts of survival. However, while in the London case this struggle tends to amplify social isolation (the argument being that one cannot 'afford' to be 'vulnerable' in a city like London), for Neapolitan immigrants it often seems to be the trigger for expanding social interactions and solidarity networks.

Notes

1 The term 'modern' ghetto is used by Wirth (1927) to distinguish contemporary Jewish immigrants' settlements in Western cities from their 'old' equivalents, namely medieval institutions used to segregate the Jews from the rest of the population. For a further distinction between the 'old' and 'new' ghetto see also Marcuse (1997).
2 Peach's critique centres in particular on Park's overall understanding of the ghetto and the ethnic enclave as two *stages* of a three-generational model (2005: 40–41): ghetto, ethnic enclave, suburb.
3 According to Wirth (1928: 284), 'the physical distance that separates these immigrant areas from that of the native population is at the same time a measure of the social distance between them and a means by which this social distance can be maintained'.
4 The term 'segregation' is generally used in its 'neutral' meaning by most urban sociologists, without any reference to 'coercion or choice', as explained by van Kempen and Özüekren (1998: 1633).
5 A term used by Massey and Denton (1989: 388–389), hyper-segregation refers to a condition often experienced by African-American groups in US cities, consisting of 'an accumulation of segregation across multiple dimensions simultaneously' which results in an unprecedented 'level of spatial isolation' among this category.
6 Principally, 'Moving to Opportunity' in the US, but also a number of similar projects in France, Finland and the Netherlands, among others.
7 A small cash fee (£10) was offered as an incentive.
8 Butler (2007), for example, warns that a distinction should be made between the 'gentrification' phenomenon and other forms of urban reconfiguration, such as 'sub-urbanization' processes which are qualitatively different from the former.
9 However, a study conducted by Atkinson (2000a: 318) shows that the displacement of former 'indigenous' inhabitants of regenerated London areas is frequently found to be obtained not only via rental and prices increases (or offers of cash money) but also by means of 'harassment, violence and intimidation'.
10 However this figure does not include immigrants who are not officially resident in Naples.
11 Figures of the Migration Observatory. Full report available at www.migratio nobservatory.ox.ac.uk/resources/briefings/migrants-in-the-uk-an-overview/.
12 This means family, friends or acquaintances who they knew in their home country before emigrating.
13 A Neapolitan expression meaning to set one's home and place of work in the same place (*puteca*, Neapolitan for *bottega*, 'shop').
14 Muslim immigrants interviewed in London said they do not practise *zakat* in the UK and that it is generally their parents' duty at home to do so.

8 Blame it on the stranger

'Us vs them'

We have arrived at the end of our journey through morality and solidarity. In this concluding chapter, we look again at the moral boundaries of our society from the standpoint of two key sociological concepts: the *outsider* and the *stranger*. A notion derived from the sociology of knowledge of Robert K. Merton, the outsider can only be defined in conjunction with its opposite, the insider. For Merton (1972: 21), insiders are 'the members of specified groups and collectivities or occupants of specified social statuses', whereas outsiders can be simply defined as 'the non-members'. This definition evidently makes every single individual belong to one of the two categories, depending on status, role and situation taken into consideration. The undeserving poor, following this definition, can be considered as those 'who are not excused' from work (Handler, 1993: 859), no matter how large this group may have become today.

In retrospect, the whole book, and the discussion we made, can be looked at as a discussion on the social, moral and spatial position kept by economic outsiders in different contexts and at different points in time. Looking back at the first chapters in the volume, we find figures of outsiders such as beggars and paupers, who were basically punished with their physical isolation from the rest of society to prevent moral and sanitary 'contamination'. Later in the book we discussed how the 'parasite', the 'welfare queen' and 'the scrounger' became the object of a *symbolic* form of ostracism occurring through the social stigmatisation of economic outsiders in the press. Eventually, we discussed how the Great Recession and restraining welfare budgets have reconfigured, once again, the moral argument against undeserving claimants and the form of *civic punishment* and exclusion from social redistribution.

This chapter is structured as follows. First a section on the latest events in Italy and Britain illustrates the impact of two different types of crisis (Brexit and the refugee crisis respectively) on the identification of new scapegoats: immigrants and refugees. The following section describes the process of scapegoating today and analyses the 'stranger' as the perfect economic scapegoat of our times. The last section of the chapter reviews the main results in the book against the background provided by Wacquant's (2009) argument on the 'survival of the fittest' and discusses the case for the disruption of solidarity in our society.

Scroungers, migrants and refugees in the aftermath of the Great Recession: is it all about money?

When former UK Prime Minister David Cameron shared his concerns about the immigration issue as something that 'boils down to one word: control', the Mediterranean migrant crisis and the Calais events of July 2015 in which at least two people died in an attempt to reach the UK from France were still a long way off. 'Brexit' – i.e. the exit of the UK from the European Union – was discussed, but by and large it was felt as an unimaginable scenario. Yet the tone of emergency in these words, pronounced during Cameron's 'Speech on Immigration' on 28 November 2014, is indicative of both the general climate surrounding the debate over immigration policy and its escalating urgency since that time. Unsurprisingly, the very word 'control' figures 17 times in Cameron's speech, a clear indication of the government's overall approach to this theme: immigration flows can and should be controlled so as to be centred ·on, in the words of Cameron, *'our* national interest'.[1] The predominance of the national interest in the Coalition's rhetoric on immigration is best illustrated by considering the relatively scant appearance of the word 'migrant' (17 times) in Cameron's speech as compared to the words 'British' (24 times) and 'Britain' (33 times).

The most striking and interesting aspect of that speech, however, is Cameron's continuous reference to the British welfare state allegedly acting as an *attracting pole* for immigrants, both working and jobless. The direct link between immigration and social policy programmes which is made in this speech is best summarised by Cameron's argument that those who deny the existence of an immigration problem in the UK 'have never waited on a social housing list'.

In addressing the immigration issue by explicitly bringing up the need to reduce the number of those coming to the UK *and* to reform the welfare sector altogether, however, Cameron's speech anticipated two of the central points in the political 'Leave' campaign of 2015–2016. First, that the main concern for both the public and the government with regard to immigration attains to the *economic* sphere, rather than its potential cultural and social implications. Second, and more specifically, the fear (or perception) that the labour market, social services and the welfare budget could become overburdened due to growing immigration.

Former UKIP leader Nigel Farage and other politicians made a clear economic argument in their Leave campaign: that the British welfare system was a strong 'incentive' for immigrants to enter the UK. Soon enough, the whole Leave campaign began to be populated by references to an apparent opposition of the native British population to 'benefit migrants' who 'have no moral right to a claim on that money', as *Telegraph* columnist Julia Hartley-Brewer maintained.[2] Another UKIP representative, Member of the European Parliament (MEP) Mike Hookem, explicitly resorted to this very dichotomy when he declared that the British welfare state has not been set up to enrich 'Gypsy Kings in Romania ... building lavish palaces funded by people in the UK working on the minimum wage'.[3] The perceived strong separation between natives and immigrants is therefore primarily to be understood in economic terms, resulting from the fear that immigrants would take over the (scarce) resources of the British population. However, these debates and the relevant moralising divisions they produce, also signal the growth of *social anxiety* increasingly determining relationships with those conceived as outsiders, be they immigrants from across the Channel or native British individuals who supposedly 'sponge off' society by undeservingly claiming social benefits.

In fact, while Cameron made explicitly clear in his speech that the British 'welfare system is like a national club', so as to underline that it is designed especially for British citizens; he also explained that 'the problem hasn't just been a simplistic one of too many people coming here; it's also been [one of] too many British people without the incentive to work because they can get a better income living on benefits.' Cameron's speech on immigration illustrates well how the current narrative around the danger associated with uncontrolled flows of immigrants coming to the UK overlaps, in a way, with the rhetoric about those who fraudulently or undeservingly or even illicitly exploit the British welfare system. This very rhetoric has only gained momentum both in the UK and in other European countries during the last few years, and in particular in its conjunction with the electoral campaign of spring 2015, featuring, among others, declarations by then UKIP leader Nigel Farage on 'the right to be concerned if a group of Romanian people suddenly moved in next door'.[4] As is the case in other parts of Europe, it is not uncommon for electoral campaigns to make explicit use of public anxiety concerning welfare abuse or an imminent 'barbarian-style invading Roma underclass' (Fekete, 2014: 62) in order to gain political consent. Take the case of the refugee crisis in Italy. The rise of asylum seekers reaching Italy by boat since 2013 is an undeniable phenomenon.

However, the sense of mounting 'emergency' often disseminated by the media can be put into perspective by looking at the real figures: arrivals in 2015 (153,842 immigrants) are in fact much lower than those recorded for 2014 (170,100).[5] Yet the alarming tones used by a number of right-wing politicians, first and foremost Lega Nord leader Matteo Salvini, depict a different reality: an incessant 'invasion' of 'fake' refugees who allegedly are not escaping war and political oppression.[6] The emphasis put on these refugees as 'economic migrants' has become central in the immigration rhetoric and is gaining consensus among the public. The argument made by Salvini and many others in the political arena is that Italy is far beyond its capacity to host the increasing number of asylum seekers, and that the state should first 'provide shelter and food to its own citizens and then give *to others* if there is any money left'.[7] This argument comes together with mounting protest and discomfort among a section of the public at the idea that refugees hosted in Italian cities, who are not entitled to work, will be eating and sleeping 'at Italians' expense',[8] a concern that inevitably echoes back to the 'idleness anxiety' of pre-industrial England.

The same argument however is also increasingly applied to other categories of migrants, among whom are the Roma people in Italy at the centre of a number of xenophobic protests over the last few years. As is the case for Britain, the core element in the attacks against immigrants is then first and foremost an economic one, although there is also the expression of concern for the social dimension of immigration, the most visible manifestation of which is the recent escalation of anti-immigration protests in the central Italian village of Gorino. Here the population raised barricades to block the arrival of 12 refugee women who were supposed to find shelter in a local hostel, and expressed anger at the prospect that their town would be invaded by 'criminality and degeneration', as one of the protesters said.

Events of this sort do not lessen the extent of solidarity actions towards refugees and migrants in Italy, or the call for a 'Christian' approach to their assistance.[9] However, the combination of economic factors (the dispersion of scant resources) and fear for social and cultural characteristics of the 'other' can be said to be the main elements of new forms of 'moral panic' around the immigration topic, both in Italy and in the UK.

Having clarified the contexts in which the latest events have been displayed, it is now worth discussing whether the exacerbation of an insider/outsider opposition narrative in the post-recession context corresponds to intensification of outsiders' scapegoating in the public arena. In order to do so we will be drawing upon a second sociological notion, i.e. the 'stranger'.

Scapegoating the 'other': the stranger

The most interesting aspect in exploring 'scapegoating' processes in society is without doubt the multifaceted nature of the concept itself. Depending on whether one looks at scapegoating from a sociological, psychological, criminological or political point of view (just to mention a few), its specific definition may assume different connotations and provoke very diverse insights. A good point of departure is the sociological notion of 'scapegoat', defined as 'the person or group that is *chosen* to bear the brunt of frustration or re-direct aggression' (Bruce and Yearley, 2006: 269, emphasis added). Even more pertinent to our discussion of this specific definition, however, is the explanation of the process itself: scapegoating practices are seen as something occurring 'when people are unable to identify the real source of their (for example, economic) problems, or having identified the source, are unable to challenge it' (ibid.).

Such a definition best summarises a fundamental aspect of our discussion: that the modern and contemporary features of scapegoating in our society are evidently less centred on its original religious dimension and increasingly more affected by societal *anxiety* concerning economic, political and social issues, welfare entitlements and immigration, among others.[10] In fact, in one of the earliest and best-known studies on scapegoating and prejudice, by social psychologist Gordon W. Allport (1954), noted that scapegoating practices cannot be exclusively explained by socio-cultural factors as they are also intrinsically and historically bound to *societal attitudes* towards what he referred to as 'psychological minorities', most notably immigrants; but undeserving welfare claimants can be easily added to this category.

In addressing the question of how society perceives and treats these socio-economic and psychological minorities, especially in times of crisis, we can turn to the argument recently formulated by Ash Amin (2012: 130) that the entire problem of immigration, community and solidarity in society is precisely a matter of our relationship with the 'stranger', with the history of Western and European social models being a history of 'withdrawal from the stranger in times of adversity and of qualified support at other times'. This argument stands as a fundamental premise in our discussion of the 'us versus them' narrative, whether it concerns immigrants or undeserving welfare claimants and seems consistent with the overall description which has been made in the book.

This connotation of the 'stranger' is indeed profoundly different from its classic conceptualisations, such as the one formulated by Bauman (1989; Bauman, 1991), for whom strangers are an 'untouchable' class, mainly characterised by its *passive* dimension, kept at the outskirts of our cities, preferably invisible to our eyes. Conversely, Amin's interpretation of the modern-era stranger is one strictly bound to *our* negative feelings towards *them* and to a distinctive *active* approach directed at 'name and shame, curtail and contain, discipline and eject, domesticate and assimilate', which is, quite paradoxically, defended in the name of a fair and 'egalitarian' way of life (2012: 122).

Such an approach is especially evident in the shift from a passive-oriented approach in our treatment of strangers towards a much more active endeavour to eliminate those deemed as constituting a threat to our society. This shift, however, is not merely a semantic one. Scapegoating in times of crisis may also have profound material repercussions, for practical steps may be taken to deal with social and economic problems for which scapegoats are blamed, as the immigration and welfare reform agenda outlined by Cameron in his speech clearly evidenced. The Gorino case in Italy and the Brexit result in the UK are possibly two fitting examples of this process, with justifications for the attack on immigration generally being associated with the safeguard of internal values, resources and national lifestyles. It is not surprising that the most recurrent arguments against today's scapegoats such as immigrants, refugees and 'undeserving' welfare claimants are based on economic justifications. These groups have frequently been the focus of public discussion over the last few years and have increasingly been perceived, both in the political arena and by the public opinion of several countries, as major 'threats' to the status quo.

If we look back to the argument made in this book, we find many examples of scapegoating practices towards the stranger. Could we deny that social anxiety over the impending arrival in English cities of a large army of a stranger, inactive rural poor – the so-called 'dangerous poor' (Morris, 2002) – at the end of 1800s was in fact a public reaction of incomprehension of economic phenomena? What was the real objective of workhouse internment if not an attempt at *disciplining and domesticating* the inactive able-bodied poor? And again, can we find a more fitting example of 'cathartic objects' of scapegoating (Gans, 1994: 272) in times of crisis than the communist parasite, the welfare queen or its British equivalent, the 'scrounger'?

Finally, it is interesting to note that although most of these scapegoating practices may be explained on economic grounds, they are generally justified with 'moralising' arguments insisting on assumed deviant traits or behaviours of the stranger (a 'welfare fraudster', a 'fake refugee', an 'immoral mother') so as to deny that the real cause of concern is essentially an economic one.

Every man for himself, or the 'survival of the fittest'

One of the main characteristics of all the episodes of 'moral panic' addressed in this book is that they came together with a number of common dynamics. First and foremost, each 'moral crisis' described in the book brought about a redefinition of the notion of deservedness and its main features, including the distinction between 'worthy' and 'unworthy' poor or claimants and the methods for distinguishing between the two. Secondly, most episodes of moral panic around poverty were similar in preparing the ground for the emergence of new legislative instruments to 'regulate' the poor and to exert surveillance over and discipline upon them. Thirdly, they often produced apparently incoherent solutions to the problem of poverty, most of the time derived from the need to combine irreconcilable ideological, normative and political approaches to the issue.

At a general level, we can say that each of these episodes – as is the case with most types of crisis – called into question the dominating poverty epistemology. In this respect the history of moral panics around poverty is undoubtedly a history of both progressive innovations and reactionary solutions to the never-ending problem of how to protect the poor by incentivising them to work.

A fascinating perspective from which we can further analyse the long-term trajectory of moralisation in the welfare state can be derived from the work of Loïc Wacquant. He postulates that the increasing emphasis on workfare and the moral argument against welfare dependency is part of a wider historical process of transformation gradually driving society towards the symbolic (and actual) punishment of the poor. In this transformation, he contends, society transitioned from a situation wherein the Keynesian-Fordist socio-economic model would guarantee solidarity and reduce inequalities to a 'neo-Darwinist' era that 'celebrates unrestrained individual responsibility' by legitimising 'collective and political irresponsibility' at the same time. The ultimate effect of this transition, Wacquant notes, is a 'struggle for [economic] life' (2009: 5–6).

Can we argue that the profound economic downturn created by the Great Recession and the latest events in Europe resulted in a new struggle of one poor against the other? Long-term transformations (such as the increasing re-enforcement of the contractual component of welfare systems) seem to validate such a view. It is undeniable, for example, that one of the effects of the deteriorating living conditions of the middle class is that the working poor are now competing to access the same resources the unemployed crave, social benefits among others. However, it would be oversimplifying to assume that solidarity as a whole is being completely disrupted in our society.

If we consider the argument made by Wacquant against the findings of this book, the continuity line he uses seems more questionable, albeit not incompatible with our own results. On the one hand, if we look at public opinions and attitudes towards poverty and deservedness in the welfare state, it cannot be said that the general trend is that of a progressive disenchantment of solidarity values among the public. Our analysis of Eurobarometer data, for example, indicates that culturalistic interpretations of poverty in Britain (poverty equals laziness or wrong individual behaviour) grew during the Great Recession, only to become less diffused in the immediate aftermath of the crisis.

The findings from our focus group experiment, conversely, show that moralistic classifications of 'deserving' and 'undeserving' poor may persist even after the crisis, although the identification of 'immigrants' and 'asylum seekers' as typical cases of welfare 'scroungers' must be noted an unprecedented trend. It is significant in this respect that the strongest reactions in our focus group discussions were expressed in regard to the theme of immigration. The frequent emergence of negative sentiments about immigrants as a category deemed 'unworthy' of receiving welfare payments is something which seems to validate Wacquant's grim prospect for a new type of struggle between different kinds of claimants. Thus while it can be said that the historical trend identified by Wacquant is by all means applicable to the findings and to the general argument of the book, the distinctive focus on episodes of moral panic around poverty provides a further fundamental lens for a full understanding of the 'ups and downs' of solidarity towards the poor in the post-industrial society. Among other things, this perspective can shed some light on the different reasons behind the exacerbation of misconceptions and myths around the undeserving poor. The perception of an invading wave of immigrants abusing the welfare system or engaging in 'welfare tourism' in their movements across Europe, for example, has certainly been amplified by the alarming tones of the media and politicians alike, especially in conjunction with political campaigns. At the same time, the moralising attacks on 'welfare mothers' dependent on benefits and accused of giving birth to children irrespective of their economic capacity to feed them, a constant element in our focus group discussions, is an expression of escalating sensationalism in the

British press since 2014. Nevertheless, in concluding this study, it is worth asking what the practical consequences of these misconceptions are on solidarity in our society – something which brings us directly to the final section of this book.

Urban coexistence: big societies and micro-neighbourhoods

Anxiety derived from the potential physical proximity with the 'dangerous poor' is a constant theme in the history of moral panic episodes in Europe. The increasing fear of 'contamination' by a part of the city's poor, for example, was typical of the Victorian age, during which increasing concern for the prospect of 'urban degeneration' phenomena only added to the diffused misconceptions of the time about poverty, let alone the stigmatising treatment of the poor. Arguably, the attribution of a deviant character to the undeserving poor is still valid today as a general trend. It is tempting in fact to analogise the Victorian anxiety for a process of urban degeneration with recent episodes of violent attacks against immigrants. The case of Gorino mentioned above is a fitting example of this mechanism, with the local population attributing their anger and protest against hosting refugees to grounds that their 'clean' town could be contaminated by criminals and degenerates.

This and similar episodes are significant indications of the progressive exacerbation of urban coexistence in society and of the fact that spatial exclusion of its members is re-emerging as a major problem in our cities. David Cameron's plea for the formation of a Big Society which could help community members in an informal but effective way could not seem more unattainable from this stance. Our interviews with immigrants confirm that in global cities like London community ties at the local level are fragmented and often only superficial. Needless to say, solidarity opportunities at the neighbourhood level are almost impossible, and young people often find themselves relying on 'micro-neighbours' – comprising their most immediate relatives, close friends and flatmates. These artificial micro-neighbours, our discussion evidenced, often function as valid alternatives to practices of mutual help and support generally found at the neighbourhood level, especially for immigrants living far from their native community.

Yet it is precisely at the neighbourhood level that we can find the remnants of solidarity and social cohesion. The description of Naples, with Piazza Garibaldi and other areas of the city centre functioning as magnets for migrants of different nationalities, is exemplifying in this respect. Here solidarity and mutual help networks are constructed through face-to-face daily practices. One could ask whether these are the last remnants of solidarity in general. With welfare systems across Europe, in Wacquant's argument, becoming increasingly more preoccupied with work incentives and controls over the behaviour of claimants, solidarity as an expression of the post-war social contract is to say the least eroded. At the same time, sympathy for the poor and for new categories of welfare claimants such as immigrants and refugees, is subject to external events, such as economic crises or political campaigns, that can alternately amplify or decrease public anxiety over 'the stranger'.

In sum, it is possible to draw a major conclusion from the study conducted in this book. The moral line that can divide deserving and undeserving poor in our society, insiders and outsiders, is under continuous evolution. Yesterday's 'worthy' poor, such as lone mothers, are today's scapegoats. At the same time, scientific accounts that aim at explaining in rigorous terms the problem of poverty and destitution can easily stumble upon moralising rationales. The recurrent re-emergence of a knowledge of poverty based on cultural explanations of this phenomenon is indicative of such possibilities, but is the recent (re)appearance of a 'biologisation of poverty' trend in social economic studies to be most worrisome? These accounts identify childhood experience of poverty and bad parenting as a major *biological factor* affecting future poor living conditions of children, indirectly pointing the finger at the responsibility of parents and their misconduct in undermining (quite deterministically) the future economic and social outcomes of their children.[11] How this approach is substantially different from the eugenic concern of Victorians over the transmission of 'degenerate' genes among the urban poor is hard to say.

Notes

1 Prime Minister's Speech held on 28 November 2014 at JCB Staffordshire (emphasis added). Full text available at www.gov.uk/government/speeches/jcb-staffordshire-prime-ministers-speech.
2 Extract from 'If David Cameron doesn't stop European migrants claiming benefits, Britain cannot stay in the EU', *Telegraph*, 9 December 2015.
3 *Express*, 5 April 2016.
4 Nigel Farage declaration available at www.ukip.org/ukip_leader_stands_by_his_assertion_that_people_have_a_right_to_be_concerned_if_a_group_of_romanians_move_in_next_door.
5 *Repubblica*, data available at www.repubblica.it/solidarieta/immigrazione/2016/01/07/news/flussi_migratori_12_mesi_di_sbarchi_in_europa-130787694/.
6 *Ansa*, 12 May 2016.
7 Extract from declaration of 5 September 2016 (emphasis added), available on Lega Nord's official webpage. http://leganord.org/notizie/le-news-2/13057-immigrati-salvini-dare-prima-a-italiani-e-poi-se-avanza-a-loro.
8 *Il Giornale*, 29 March 2016.
9 A Catholic priest has recently hit the headlines for saying during a sermon that 'you are either Salvini supporters, or you are Christian *Ansa*, 8 November 2016, available at www.ansa.it/english/news/politics/2016/11/08/salvini-asks-removal-of-catholic-priest_1347da7a-4ba5-45e2-82fb-dc680583ff4e.html.
10 It is a truism acknowledged in most studies, however, that even the utmost form of religious scapegoating, i.e. anti-Semitism, contained a strong economic component.
11 A recent report from an Independent Review on Poverty and Life Chances commissioned by the British government made the case for the interruption of 'the intergenerational cycle of disadvantage' based on a similar explanation (Field, 2010).

References

Aaronson, M. N. (1996). Scapegoating the poor: welfare reform all over again and the undermining of democratic citizenship. *Hastings Women's Law Journal*, 7, 213–256.

Abel-Smith, B. (1992). The Beveridge report: its origins and outcomes. *International Social Security Review*, 45(1–2), 5–16.

Abbott, E. (1938). Is there a legal right to relief? *Social Service Review*, 12(2), 260–275.

Albini, G. (2002). *Carità e governo delle povertà: secoli XII–XV*. Milano: Unicopli.

Albrow, M. (2012). Big Society as a rhetorical intervention. In A. Ishkanian and S. Szreter *The Big Society Debate: A New Agenda for Social Welfare?* Cheltenham: Edward Elgar.

Alcock, T. (1752). *Observations on the Defects of the Poor Laws, and on the Causes and Consequences of the Great Increase and Burden of the Poor*. London and Oxford: Baldwin and Clements.

Aldrete, G. S. (1994). *Daily Life in the Roman City: Rome, Pompeii and Ostia*. Westport, CT and London: Greenwood.

Allport, G. W. (1954). *The Nature of Prejudice*. Reading: Addison-Wesley.

Althusser, L. (2006). Ideology and ideological state apparatuses (notes towards an investigation). In A. Sharma and A. Gupta (eds) *The Anthropology of the State: A Reader*. Malden, MA: Blackwell.

Altreiter, C., and Leibetseder, B. (2015). Constructing Inequality: Deserving and Undeserving Clients in Austrian Social Assistance Offices. *Journal of Social Policy*, 44(1), 127–145.

Amin, A. (2012). *Land of Strangers*. Cambridge: Polity Press.

Applebaum, L. D. (2001). The influence of perceived deservingness on policy decisions regarding aid to the poor. *Political Psychology*, 22(3), 419–442.

Ascoli, U., and Pavolini, E. (eds) (2015). *The Italian Welfare State in a European Perspective: A Comparative Analysis*. Bristol: Policy Press.

Atkinson, R. (2000a). The hidden costs of gentrification: displacement in central London. *Journal of Housing and the Built Environment*, 15(4), 307–326.

Atkinson, R. (2000b). Measuring gentrification and displacement in Greater London. *Urban Studies*, 37(1), 149–165.

Atkinson, R., and Bridge, G. (eds) (2005). *Gentrification in a Global Context*. London: Routledge.

Aydelotte, F. (1913). *Elizabethan Rogues and Vagabonds*. Oxford: Clarendon.

Bagnasco, A., and Le Galés, P. (2000). 'Introduction. European cities: local societies and collective actors. Cities in Contemporary Europe'. In A. Bagnasco and P. Le Galés (eds) *Cities in Contemporary Europe*. Cambridge: Cambridge University Press.

Baldwin, P. (1990). *The Politics of Social Solidarity: Class Bases of the European Welfare State.* Cambridge: Cambridge University Press.

Banfield, E. C. (1958). *The Moral Basis of a Backward Society.* New York: The Free Press.

Bayer, P., Ross, S., and Topa, G. (2004). Place of work and place of residence: informal hiring networks and labor market outcomes. Economics Working Papers 2004–2007, University of Connecticut.

Bauman, Z. (1989). *Modernity and the Holocaust.* Oxford: Blackwell.

Bauman, Z. (1991). *Modernity and Ambivalence.* Cambridge: Polity Press.

Beaumont, J. (2006). London: deprivation, social isolation and regeneration. In S. Musterd, A. Murie, and C. Kesteloot (eds) *Neighbourhoods of Poverty: Urban Social Exclusion and Integration in Europe.* Basingstoke: Palgrave Macmillan.

Becchi, A. (1989). Napoli contro Napoli. Città come economia e città come potere. *Meridiana*, 5, 143–167.

Beermann, R. (1964). Soviet and Russian anti-parasite laws. *Soviet Studies*, 15(4), 420–429.

Beier, A. L. (1974). Vagrants and the social order in Elizabethan England. *Past and Present*, 64, 3–29.

Beier, A. L. (1985). *Masterless Men: The Vagrancy Problem in England 1560–1640.* London: Methuen.

Bentham, J. (1796) [2001]. *Writings on the Poor Laws.* Oxford: Oxford University Press.

Bentham, J. (1778). *The Works of Jeremy Bentham.* Edinburgh: William Tait.

Beresford, P. (2016). Presenting welfare reform: poverty porn, telling sad stories or achieving change? *Disability and Society*, 31(3), 421–425.

Berger, P. L., and Luckmann, T. (1967). *The Social Construction of Reality: A Treatise in the Sociology of Knowledge.* London: Penguin.

Berry, C. (2016). *Austerity Politics and UK Economic Policy.* London: Palgrave Macmillan.

Bianchi, F., and Słoń, M. (2006). Le riforme ospedaliere del Quattrocento in Italia e nell'Europa centrale. *Ricerche di storia sociale e religiosa*, 35, 7–45.

Black, C. (2001). *Early Modern Italy: A Social History.* London: Routledge.

Bolis, G. (1871). *La polizia e le classi pericolose della società.* Modena: Nicola Zanichelli.

Bonnell, V. E. (1997). *Iconography of Power: Soviet Political Posters under Lenin and Stalin.* Berkeley: University of California Press.

Booth, C. (1903). *Life and Labour of the People in London.* London: Macmillan.

Borzaga, C. (2004). From suffocation to re-emergence: the evolution of the Italian third sector. In A. Evers and J.-L. Laville (eds) *The Third Sector in Europe.* Cheltenham: Edward Elgar.

Bosanquet, B. (1910). Charity organization and the majority report. *International Journal of Ethics*, 20(4), 395–408.

Brewer, M., Browne, J., Hood, A., Joyce, R., and Sibieta, L. (2013). The short-and medium-term impacts of the recession on the UK income distribution. *Fiscal Studies*, 34(2), 179–201.

Brimicombe, A. J. (2007). Ethnicity, religion, and residential segregation in London: evidence from a computational typology of minority communities. *Environment and Planning B: Planning and Design*, 34(5), 884–904.

Brooks, C., and Manza, J. (2006). Why do welfare states persist? *Journal of Politics*, 68(4), 816–827.

Bruce, S., and Yearley, S. (2006). *The Sage Dictionary of Sociology.* London: Sage.

Brundage, A. (2002). *The English Poor Laws, 1700–1930.* Basingstoke: Palgrave Macmillan.

Burgess, E. W. (1928). Residential segregation in American cities. *Annals of the American Academy of Political and Social Science,* 140, 105–115.

Burgess, S., Wilson, D., and Lupton, R. (2005). Parallel lives? Ethnic segregation in schools and neighbourhoods. *Urban studies,* 42(7), 1027–1056.

Burke, E. (1791). On the rupture of the negotiation. the terms of peace proposed; and the resources of the country. In *The Works of Edmund Burke.* Boston: Little & Brown.

Burn, R. (1764). *The History of the Poor Laws: With Observations.* London: Woodfall and Strahan.

Burnett, J. (1994). *Idle Hands. The Experience of Unemployment, 1790–1990.* London and New York: Routledge.

Butler, T. (2003). Living in the bubble: gentrification and its 'others' in North London. *Urban Studies,* 40(12), 2469–2486.

Butler, T. (2007). Re-urbanizing London Docklands: gentrification, suburbanization or new urbanism? *International Journal of Urban and Regional Research,* 31(4), 759–781.

Butler, T., and Lees, L. (2006). Super-gentrification in Barnsbury, London: globalization and gentrifying global elites at the neighbourhood level. *Transactions of the Institute of British Geographers,* 31(4), 467–487.

Callum, D. R. (1995). Soviet society and law: the history of the legal campaign to enforce the constitutional duty to work. PhD thesis, University of Glasgow.

Camera deiDeputati del ParlamentoItaliano (1913). *Discorsi Parlamentari di Silvio Spaventa.* Roma: Tipografia della Camera dei Deputati.

Canciullo, G. (2010). Accattoni. L'Albergo Ventimigliano di Catania tra idee, lessico e rappresentazioni. *Studi storici,* 51(1), 239–259.

Carey, M. A., and Asbury, J. E. (2012). *Focus Group Research.* Abingdon: Routledge.

Carroll, W. C. (1996). *Fat King, Lean Beggar: Representations of Poverty in the Age of Shakespeare.* Ithaca, NY: Cornell University Press.

Cassata, F. (2011). *Building the New Man: Eugenics, Racial Science and Genetics in Twentieth-Century Italy.* Budapest and New York: Central European University Press.

Castel, R. (2003). *From Manual Workers to Wage Laborers: Transformation of the Social Question.* London: Transaction.

Censis (2012). *Gli scenari del welfare. Le nuove tutele oltre la crisi.* Milano: Franco Angeli.

Chambliss, W. J. (1964). A sociological analysis of the law of vagrancy. *Social Problems,* 12(1), 67–77.

Chambliss, W. J. (2004). A sociological analysis of the law of vagrancy. In A. K. Stout, R. A. Dello Buono, and W. J. Chambliss (eds) *Social Problems, Law, and Society.* Lanham, MD: Rowman & Littlefield.

Charlesworth, L. (2012). Big society, legal structures, poor law and the myth of a voluntary society. In A. Ishkanian, and S. Szreter, (eds). *The Big Society Debate: A New Agenda for Social Policy?* Cheltenham: Edward Elgar.

Cheshire, P. (2007). *Segregated Neighbourhoods and Mixed Communities: A Critical Analysis.* York: Joseph Rowntree Foundation.

Chunn, D. E., and Gavigan, S. A. (2004). Welfare law, welfare fraud, and the moral regulation of the 'never deserving' poor. *Social and Legal Studies,* 13(2), 219–243.

Ciucci, G. (1995). Premessa. In A. Guerra, E. Molteni, and P. Nicoloso (eds) *Il trionfo della miseria. gli alberghi dei poveri di Genova, Palermo e Napoli*. Milano: Electa.

Ciuffetti, A. (2004). *Difesa sociale. povertà, assistenza e controllo in Italia: XVI–XX secolo* (Vol. 3). Perugia: Morlacchi Editore.

Clarke, J., and Cochrane, A. (1998). The social construction of social problems. In E. Saraga (ed.) *Embodying the Social: Constructions of Difference*. London: Routledge.

Clasen, J., and Clegg, D. (2007). Levels and levers of conditionality. measuring change within welfare states. In J. Clasen and N. A. Siegel (eds) *Investigating Welfare State Change: The 'Dependent Variable Problem' in Comparative Analyses*. Cheltenham: Edward Elgar.

Clawson, R. A., and Trice, R. (2000). Poverty as we know it: media portrayals of the poor. *Public Opinion Quarterly*, 64(1), 53–64.

Clery, E. (2012). Welfare: are tough times affecting attitudes to welfare? In A. Park, E. Clery, J. Curtice, M. Phillips, and D. Utting (eds) *British Social Attitudes: The 29th Report*. London: NatCen Social Research.

Coats, A. W. (1958). Changing attitudes to labour in the mid-eighteenth century. *Economic History Review*, 11(1), 35–51.

Coats, A. W. (1976). The relief of poverty, attitudes to labour, and economic change in England, 1660–1782, prepared for the Sixth Meeting of the International Institute of Economic History 'Francesco Datini' at Prato, April 1974.

Cohen, S. (1972) [2002]. *Folk Devils and Moral Panics: The Creation of the Mods and the Rockers*. Abingdon: Routledge.

Colwill, J. (1994). Beveridge, women and the welfare state. *Critical Social Policy*, 14(41), 53–78.

Comte, A. (1851) [1973]. *The System of Positive Polity: Treatise on Sociology Instituting the Religion of Humanity*. New York: Burt Franklin.

Corbett, S., and Walker, A. (2013). The big society: rediscovery of 'the social' or rhetorical fig-leaf for neo-liberalism? *Critical Social Policy*, 33(3), 451–472.

Coser, L. A. (1965). The sociology of poverty: to the memory of Georg Simmel. *Social Problems*, 13(2), 140–148.

Crowther, M. A. (1981). *The Workhouse System: The history of an English Social Institution*. Cambridge: Cambridge University Press.

D'Andrea, D. (2003). Italy: the case of Treviso. In T. M. Safley (ed.) *The Reformation of Charity: The Secular and the Religious in Early Modern Poor Relief*. Boston: Brill.

Da Passano, M. (2004). Il vagabondaggio nell'Italia dell'ottocento. *Acta Histriae*, 12(1), 52–92.

Darwin, C. (1859) [2005]. *On the Origin of the Species by Natural Selection*. London and New York: Routledge.

Datta, A. (2011). Translocal Geographies of London: Belonging and 'Otherness' among Polish Migrants after 2004. In K. Brickell and A. Datta (eds). *Translocal Geographies*. Farnham: Ashgate.

Davies, J. S., and Pill, M. (2012). Empowerment or abandonment? Prospects for neighbourhood revitalization under the big society. *Public Money and Management*, 32(3), 193–200.

De Acosta, M. (1997). Single mothers in the USA: unsupported workers and mothers. In S. Duncan and R. Edwards (eds) *Single Mothers in International Context: Mothers or Workers?* London and New York: Routledge.

De Filippo, E., Diana, P., Ferrara, R., and Forcellati, L. (2010). Alcuni aspetti dell'integrazione degli immigrati nella provincia di Napoli. *Rivista Italiana di Economia Demografia e Statistica*, 64(1–2), 95–102.

De Gerando, J. M. (1832). *The Visitor of the Poor*. Boston: Hilliard, Gray, Little, and Wilkins.

De Grazia, V. (1992). *How Fascism Ruled Women: Italy, 1922–1945*. Berkeley and Los Angeles: University of California Press.

Deacon, A. (1978). The scrounging controversy: public attitudes towards the unemployed in contemporary Britain. *Social and Economic Administration*, 12(2), 120–135.

Deacon, A., and Bradshaw, J. (1983). *Reserved for the Poor: The Means Test in British Social Policy*. Oxford: Blackwell and Robertson.

Deacon, A., and Patrick, R. (2011). A new welfare settlement? The Coalition government and welfare-to-work. In H. Bochel (ed.) *The Conservative Party and Social Policy*. Bristol: Policy Press.

Dean, M. (1991). *The Constitution of Poverty*. New York and London: Routledge.

Defoe, D. (1704). *Giving Alms No Charity*. London: Booksellers of London and Westminster.

Dendy, H. (1893). The industrial residuum. *Economic Journal*, 3(12), 600–616.

Dey, H. W. (2008). Diaconiae, xenodochia, hospitalia and monasteries:'social security' and the meaning of monasticism in early medieval Rome. *Early Medieval Europe*, 16(4), 398–422.

Dines, N. (2003). Urban renewal, immigration, and contested claims to public space: the case of Piazza Garibaldi in Naples. *GeoJournal*, 58(2–3), 177–188.

Dines, N. (2012). *Tuff City: Urban Change and Contested Space in Central Naples*. New York: Berghahn.

Dominelli, L. (1988). Thatcher's attack on social security: restructuring social control. *Critical Social Policy*, 8(23), 46–61.

Dorey, P. (2015). Policy responses in Britain and the economic crisis: the failure of social democracy? In S. Romano and G. Punziano (eds) *The European Social Model Adrift: Europe, Social Cohesion, and the Economic Crisis*. Farnham: Ashgate.

Driver, F. (1993) [2004]. *Power and Pauperism: The Workhouse System, 1834–1884*. Cambridge: Cambridge University Press.

Dunkling, P. (1982). *The Crisis of the Old Poor Law in England, 1795–1834: An Interpretive Essay*. New York: Garland.

Dunning, R. D. (1698). *Bread for the poor, or, A method shewing how the poor may be maintained and duly provided for in a far more plentiful and yet cheaper manner than now they are without waste or want*. Exeter: Samuel Darker.

Dziewiecka-Bokun, L. (2000). Poverty and the poor in Central and Eastern Europe. In D. Gordon and P. Townsend (eds) *Breadline Europe: The Measurement of Poverty*. Bristol: Policy Press.

Eden, F. M. (1797). *The State of the Poor*. London: J. Davies.

Edsall, N. C. (1971). *The Anti-Poor Law Movement, 1834–44*. Manchester: Manchester University Press.

Ellis, M., Wright, R., and Parks, V. (2004). Work together, live apart? Geographies of racial and ethnic segregation at home and at work. *Annals of the Association of American Geographers*, 94(3), 620–637.

Englander, D. (1998). *Poverty and Poor Law Reform in 19th Century Britain, 1834–1914*. London and New York: Longman.

Esping-Andersen, G. (1990). *The Three Worlds of Welfare Capitalism*. Princeton: Princeton University Press.

Esping-Andersen, G. (1999). *Social Foundations of Postindustrial Economies*. Oxford: Oxford University Press.

Farrell-Vinay, G. (1989). The old charities and the new state: structures and problems of welfare in Italy (1860–1890). Doctoral thesis, University of Edinburgh.

Fatica, M. (1982). La regolarizzazione dei mendicanti attraverso il lavoro: l'Ospizio dei poveri di Modena nel Settecento. *Studi storici*, 23(4), 757–782.

Fekete, L. (2014). Europe against the Roma. *Race and Class*, 55(3), 60–70.

Ferragina, E. (2009). The never-ending debate about the moral basis of a backward society: Banfield and 'amoral familism'. *Journal of Anthropological Society of Oxford*, 1(2), 141–160.

Ferrera, M. (1984). *Il Welfare State in Italia: sviluppo e crisi in prospettiva comparata*. Bologna: Mulino.

Ferrera, M. (1996). The southern model of welfare in social Europe. *Journal of European Social Policy*, 6(1), 17–37.

Ferrera, M. (1997). The uncertain future of the Italian welfare state, *West European Politics*, 20(1), 231–249.

Ferrera, M. (ed.) (2005). *Welfare State Reform in Southern Europe: Fighting Poverty and Social Exclusion in Italy, Spain, Portugal and Greece*. London and New York: Routledge.

Field, F. (2010). *The Foundation Years: Preventing Poor Children Becoming Poor Adults*. London: HM Government.

Finlayson, G. B. (1994). *Citizen, State, and Social Welfare in Britain 1830–1990*. Oxford: Clarendon.

Finney, N., and Simpson, L. (2009). *'Sleepwalking to segregation'? Challenging Myths about Race and Migration*. Bristol: Policy Press.

Fiori, A. (2005). *Poveri, opera pie e assistenza. Dall'Unità al fascismo*. Roma: Edizioni Studium.

Fitzpatrick, S. (2006). Social parasites: how tramps, idle youth, and busy entrepreneurs impeded the Soviet march to communism. *Cahiers du monde russe*, 47, 377–408.

Fitzpatrick, T., Kwon, H. J., Manning, N., Midgley, J., and Pascall, G. (2006). *International Encyclopedia of Social Policy*. London: Routledge.

Fletcher, D. (2015). Workfare: a blast from the past? Contemporary work conditionality for the unemployed in historical perspective. *Social Policy and Society*, 14(3), 329–339.

Flora, P., and Heidenheimer, A. J. (eds). (1976) [2009]. *The Development of Welfare States in Europe and America*. New Brunswick, NJ: Transaction.

Flora, P. (1981). Solution of source of crises? The welfare state in historical perspective. In W. J. Mommsen (ed.) *The Emergence of the Welfare State in Britain and Germany*. London: Croom Helm.

Fontaine, L. (2014). *The Moral Economy: Poverty, Credit, and Trust in Early Modern Europe*. New York: Cambridge University Press.

Foucault, M. (1977). *Discipline and Punish: The Birth of the Prison*. New York: Vintage.

Frampton, K. (1979). The status of man and the status of his objects: a reading of the human condition. In K. M. Hays (ed.) *Architecture Theory since 1968*. Cambridge and London: MIT Press.

Fraser, D. (1973). *The Evolution of the British Welfare State*. Basingstoke: Palgrave Macmillan.

Fraser, D. (1976). *The New Poor Law in the Nineteenth Century.* London and Basingstoke: Macmillan.

Fraser, N., and Gordon, L. (1994). 'Dependency' demystified: inscriptions of power in a keyword of the welfare state. *Social Politics: International Studies in Gender, State and Society,* 1(1), 4–31.

Freeden, M. (1979). Eugenics and progressive thought: a study in ideological affinity. *Historical Journal,* 22(03), 645–671.

Frey, R. G., and Morris, C. W. (1993). *Value, Welfare, and Morality.* Cambridge: Cambridge University Press.

Frost, F. J. (1964). Pericles, Thucydides, son of Melesias, and Athenian politics before the war. *Historia: Zeitschrift für Alte Geschichte,* 13(4), 385–399.

Fuchs, C. (2011). *Foundations of Critical Media and Information Studies.* Abingdon: Routledge.

Galton, F. (1904). Eugenics: Its definition, scope, and aims. *American Journal of Sociology,* 10(1), 1–25.

Gambardella, D., and Morlicchio, E. (2005). *Familismo forzato. Scambi di risorse e coabitazione nelle famiglie povere a Napoli.* Roma: Carocci.

Gamson, W. A., Croteau, D., Hoynes, W., and Sasson, T. (1992). Media images and the social construction of reality. *Annual Review of Sociology,* 18, 373–393.

Gans, H. J. (1994). Positive functions of the undeserving poor: uses of the underclass in America. *Politics and Society,* 22(3), 269–283.

Garland, C. (2014). Framing the poor: media illiteracy, stereotyping, and contextual fallacy to spin the crisis. *Triple C: Communication, Capitalism and Critique. Open Access Journal for a Global Sustainable Information Society,* 13(1), 5–10.

Galston, W. A., and Hoffenberg, P. H. (eds) (2010). *Poverty and Morality: Religious and Secular Perspectives.* Cambridge: Cambridge University Press.

Garnsey, P. (1988). *Famine and Food Supply in the Graeco-Roman World: Responses to Risk and Crisis.* Cambridge and New York: Cambridge University Press.

Garthwaite, K. (2014). Fear of the brown envelope: exploring welfare reform with long-term sickness benefits recipients. *Social Policy and Administration,* 48(7), 782–798.

Geremek, B. (1987). *The Margins of Society in Late Medieval Paris.* Cambridge: Cambridge University Press.

Geremek, B. (1994). *Poverty: A History.* Oxford: Blackwell.

Gervasoni, M. (1997). 'Cultura della degenerazione' tra socialismo e criminologia alla fine dell'Ottocento in Italia. *Studi storici,* 38(4), 1087–1119.

Gilbert, P. (2009). Social stakes of urban renewal: recent French housing policy. *Building Research and Information,* 37(5–6), 638–648.

Gilens, M. (1996). Race and poverty in America: public misperceptions and the American news media. *Public Opinion Quarterly,* 60(4), 515–541.

Gilliam, F. (1999). The 'welfare queen' experiment: how viewers react to images of African-American mothers on welfare. *Nieman Reports: The Nieman Foundation for Journalism at Harvard University,* 53(2). UCLA: Center for Communications and Community. Available at http://escholarship.org/uc/item/17m7r1rq.

Glass, R. (1964). Aspects of Change. In J. Brown-Saracino (ed.) *The Gentrification Debates: A Reader.* Abingdon: Routledge.

Glotz, G. (1926). *Ancient Greece at Work: An Economic History of Greece from the Homeric Period to the Roman Conquest.* New York: Barnes & Noble.

Goffman, E. (1963). *Stigma: Notes on the Management of Spoiled Identity.* Englewood Cliffs, NJ: Prentice Hall.

Golding, P., and Middleton, S. (1979). Making claims: news media and the welfare state. *Media Culture Society*, 1(5), 5–21.

Golding, P., and Middleton, S. (1982). *Images of Welfare: Press and Public Attitudes to Poverty*. Oxford: Robertson.

Gordon, L. (1990). The new feminist scholarship on the welfare state. In L. Gordon (ed.) *Women, the State and Welfare*. Madison: University of Wisconsin Press.

Gordon, L. (1992). Social insurance and public assistance: the influence of gender in welfare thought in the United States, 1890–1935. *American Historical Review*, 97(1), 19–54.

Gordon, L. (2001). Who deserves help? Who must provide? *Annals of the American Academy of Political and Social Science*, 577(1), 12–25.

Gough, I. (2001). Social assistance regimes: a cluster analysis. *Journal of European Social Policy*, 11(2), 165–170.

Goodin, R. E. (1985). *Protecting the Vulnerable: A Re-Analysis of Our Social Responsibilities*. Chicago and London: University of Chicago Press.

Goodin, R. E. (1988). *Reasons for Welfare: The Political Theory of the Welfare State*. Princeton: Princeton University Press.

Goodin, R. E., and Le Grand, J. (eds) (1999). *Not Only the Poor: The Middle Classes and the Welfare State*. London and New York: Routledge.

Gorsky, M. (1998a). Mutual aid and civil society: friendly societies in nineteenth century Bristol. *Urban History*, 25(03), 302–322.

Gorsky, M. (1998b). The growth and distribution of English friendly societies in the early nineteenth century. *Economic History Review*, 51(3), 489–511.

Granick, D. (1987). *Job Rights in the Soviet Union: Their Consequences*. Cambridge: Cambridge University Press.

Grell, O. P., Cunningham, A., and Arrizabalaga, J. (1999). *Health Care and Poor Relief in Counter-Reformation Europe*. London and New York: Routledge.

Guerra, E. (1995). L'albergo dei poveri di Genova. In A. Guerra, E. Molteni, and P. Nicoloso (eds) *Il trionfo della miseria. Gli alberghi dei poveri di Genova, Palermo e Napoli*. Milano: Electa.

Hall, S. (1980). Encoding-decoding. In S. Hall, D. Hobson, A. Lowe, and P. Willis (eds) *Culture, Media, Language*. Birmingham: Centre for Contemporary Cultural Studies.

Hamnett, C. (2003). *Unequal City: London in the Global Arena*. Abingdon: Routledge.

Hancock, A. M. (2004). *The Politics of Disgust: The Public Identity of the Welfare Queen*. New York and London: New York University Press.

Hancock, L., and Mooney, G. (2013). 'Welfare ghettos' and the 'broken society': Territorial stigmatization in the contemporary UK. *Housing, Theory and Society*, 30(1), 46–64.

Handler, J. F. (1993). Two years and you're out. *Connecticut Law Review*, 26, 857–869.

Handler, J. F., and Hasenfeld, Y. (1991). *The Moral Construction of Poverty: Welfare Reform in America*. London: Sage.

Harney, N. D. (2011). Accounting for African migrants in Naples, Italy. *Critical Perspectives on Accounting*, 22(7), 644–653.

Harp, G. J. (1995). *Positivist Republic: Auguste Comte and the Reconstruction of American Liberalism, 1865–1920*. University Park: Pennsylvanian State University Press.

Harrington, M. (1962). *The Other America: Poverty in the United States*. New York: Touchstone.

Harris, J. (1990). Enterprise and welfare states: a comparative perspective. *Transactions of the Royal Historical Society*, 40, 175–195.

Harrison, M., and Hemingway, L. (2014). Social policy and the new behaviourism: towards a more excluding society. In M. Harrison and T. Sanders (eds) *Social Policies and Social Control: New Perspectives on the 'Not-So-Big Society'*. Bristol: Policy Press.

Harrison, M., and Sanders, T. (eds) (2014). *Social Policies and Social Control: New Perspectives on the 'Not-So-Big Society'*. Bristol: Policy Press.

Haskell, H. J. (1939) [2009]. *The New Deal in Old Rome: How Government in the Ancient World Tried to Deal with Modern Problems*. New York: Knopf.

Hatcher, J. (1994). England in the aftermath of the Black Death. *Past and Present*, 144, 3–35.

Häussermann, H. (2005). The end of the European City? *European Review*, 13(02), 237–249.

Häussermann, H., and Haila, A. (2005). The European city: a conceptual framework and normative project. In Y. Kazepov (ed.) *Cities of Europe: Changing Contexts, Local Arrangements, and the Challenge to Urban Cohesion*. Malden, MA and Oxford: Blackwell.

Hayek, F. A. (1944) [2014]. *The Road to Serfdom: Text and Documents. The Definitive Edition* (ed.) B. Caldwell. Abingdon: Routledge.

Hayek, F. A. (1960). *The Constitution of Liberty*. London: Routledge & Kegan Paul.

Hayek, F. A. (1974). *Law, Legislation and Liberty*. London: Routledge & Kegan Paul.

Hemerijck, A. (2013). *Changing Welfare States*. Oxford: Oxford University Press.

Herrup, C. B. (1985). Law and Morality in Seventeenth-Century England. *Past and Present*, (106), 102–123.

Hicks, A. M. (1999). *Social Democracy and Welfare Capitalism: A Century of Income Security Politics*. New York: Cornell University Press.

Higgins, P., Campanera, J., and Nobajas, A. (2014). Quality of life and spatial inequality in London. *European Urban and Regional Studies*, 21(1), 42–59.

Hills, J. (2015). *Good Times, Bad Times: The Welfare Myth of Them and Us*. Bristol: Policy Press.

Hilton, M., Crowson, N., Mouhot, J. F., and McKay, J. (2012). *A Historical Guide to NGOs in Britain: Charities, Civil Society and the Voluntary Sector since 1945*. Basingstoke: Palgrave Macmillan.

Himmelfarb, G. (1991). *Poverty and Compassion: The Moral Imagination of the Late Victorians*. New York: Vintage.

Hug, T. B. (2009). *Impostures in Early Modern England: Representations and Perceptions of Fraudulent Identities*. Manchester: Manchester University Press.

Humphreys, R. (2001). *Poor Relief and Charity 1869–1945: The London Charity Organisation Society*. Basingstoke: Palgrave Macmillan.

Huws, U. (2015). Saints and sinners: lessons about work from daytime TV. *International Journal of Media and Cultural Politics*, 11(2), 143–163.

Istat (2014). *Generazioni a Confronto. Come Cambiano i Percorsi Verso la Vita Adulta*. Roma: Istituto nazionale di statistica.

Jacobs, K. (2015). The allure of the 'big society': conveying authority in an era of uncertainty. *Housing, Theory and Society*, 32(1), 25–38.

Jacobs, K., and Manzi, T. (2013). New localism, old retrenchment: The 'big society', housing policy and the politics of welfare reform. *Housing, Theory and Society*, 30(1), 29–45.

Jahoda, M., Lazarsfeld, P. F., and Zeisel, H. (1971). *Marienthal: The Sociography of an Unemployed Village.* New York: Aldine-Atherton.

Jensen, T. (2014). Welfare commonsense, poverty porn and doxosophy. *Sociological Research Online,* 19(3), 3.

Johnston, R., Forrest, J., and Poulsen, M. (2002a). Are there ethnic enclaves/ghettos in English cities? *Urban Studies,* 39(4), 591–618.

Johnston, R., Forrest, J., and Poulsen, M. (2002b). The ethnic geography of Ethni-Cities: the 'American model' and residential concentration in London. *Ethnicities,* 2(2), 209–235.

Johnston, R., Poulsen, M., and Forrest, J. (2007). The geography of ethnic residential segregation: a comparative study of five countries. *Annals of the Association of American Geographers,* 97(4), 713–738.

Jones, A. H. M. (1952). The economic basis of the Athenian democracy. *Past and Present,* 1, 13–31.

Jones, C., and Novak, T. (1999). *Poverty, Welfare and the Disciplinary State.* London and New York: Routledge.

Jones, G. S. (1971). *Outcast London: A Study in the Relationship between Classes in Victorian Society.* Oxford: Oxford University Press.

Jones, P. (1997). *The Italian City-State: From Commune to Signoria.* Oxford: Oxford University Press.

Jordan, S. (2003). *The Anxieties of Idleness: Idleness in Eighteenth-Century British Literature and Culture.* Lewisburg, PA: Bucknell University Press.

Jütte, R. (1994). *Poverty and Deviance in Early Modern Europe.* Cambridge: Cambridge University Press.

Iarskaia-Smirnova, E., and Romanov, P. (2014). Heroes and spongers: the iconography of disability in Soviet posters and films. In M. Rasell and E. Iarskaia-Smirnova (eds) *Disability in Eastern Europe and the Former Soviet Union: History, Policy and Everyday Life.* Abingdon: Routledge.

Kahl, S. (2005). The religious roots of modern poverty policy: Catholic, Lutheran, and Reformed Protestant traditions compared. *European Journal of Sociology/Archives Européennes de Sociologie/Europäisches Archiv für Soziologie,* 46(1), 91–126.

Kamberelis, G., and Dimitriadis, G. (2013). *Focus Groups: From Structured Interviews to Collective Conversations.* Abingdon: Routledge.

Katz, M. B. (1983). *Poverty and Policy in American History.* New York: Academic Press.

Katz, M. B. (1990) [2013]. *The Undeserving Poor: America's Enduring Confrontation with Poverty.* Oxford: Oxford University Press.

Kazepov, Y. (2015). Italian Social Assistance in the European Context: Residual innovation and uncertain futures. In U. Ascoli and E. Pavolini (eds) *The Italian Welfare State in a European Perspective: A Comparative Analysis.* Bristol: Policy Press.

Kleinman, A., and Kleinman, J. (1996). The appeal of experience: the dismay of images: cultural appropriations of suffering in our times. *Daedalus,* 125(1), 1–23.

Kohli, M., and Albertini, M. (2008). The family as a source of support for adult children's own family projects: European varieties. In C. Saraceno (ed.) *Families, Ageing and Social Policy: Intergenerational Solidarity in European Welfare States.* Cheltenham: Edward Elgar.

Kornai, J. (1992). *The Socialist System: The Political Economy of Communism.* Oxford: Oxford University Press.

Laino, G. (2014). Territorializzazione Delle Emergenze Nell'area Napoletana Fra Crisi Strutturale E Forme Di Resilienza, paper presented at the XXXV Conferenza Italiana di Scienze Regionali, Padova, 11–13 September.

Leitner, S. (2003). Varieties of familialism: the caring function of the family in comparative perspective. *European Societies*, 5(4), 353–375.

Law, S. A. (1983). Women, work, welfare, and the preservation of patriarchy. *University of Pennsylvania Law Review*, 131(6), 1249–1339.

Ledger, S. (1995). In darkest england: the terror of degeneration in 'fin de siècle' Britain. *Literature and History*, 4(2), 71.

Leibfried, S. (1993). Towards a European welfare state? In C. Jones (ed.) *New Perspectives on the Welfare State*. London: Routledge.

Lees, L. (2000). A reappraisal of gentrification: towards a 'geography of gentrification'. *Progress in Human Geography*, 24(3), 389–408.

Lees, L., Slater, T., and Wyly, E. (2008). *Gentrification*. Abingdon: Routledge.

Lees, L. H. (1998). *The Solidarities of Strangers: The English Poor Laws and the People, 1700–1948*. Cambridge: Cambridge University Press.

Leiby, J. (1985). Moral foundations of social welfare and social work: a historical view. *Social Work*, 30(4), 323–330.

Lenzer, G. (ed.) (1975). *Auguste Comte and Positivism: The Essential Writings*. New York: Harper.

Leonard, T. C. (2005). Retrospectives: eugenics and economics in the progressive era. *Journal of Economic Perspectives*, 19(4), 207–224.

Leonardi, R. (1995). Regional development in Italy: social capital and the Mezzogiorno. *Oxford Review of Economic Policy*, 11(2), 165–179.

Levenstein, L. (2004). Deserving/undeserving poor. In G. Mink and A. O'Connor (eds) *Poverty in the United States: An Encyclopedia of History, Politics, and Policy*. Santa Barbara, CA: ABC-CLIO.

Lévi-Strauss, C. (1950). *Introduction to the Work of Marcel Mauss*. London: Routledge & Kegan Paul.

Lewis, D. M. (1992). The Thirty Years' Peace. In D. M. Lewis, J. Boardman, J. K. Davies, and M. Ostwald (eds) *The Cambridge Ancient History. Vol. 5: The Fifth Century BC*. Cambridge: Cambridge University Press.

Lewis, J. (1995). *The Voluntary Sector, the State and Social Work in Britain*. Aldershot: Edward Elgar.

Lewis, O. (1959). *Five Families: Mexican Case Studies in the Culture of Poverty*. New York: Basic Books.

Lipman, P. (2011). Contesting the city: neoliberal urbanism and the cultural politics of education reform in Chicago. *Discourse: Studies in the Cultural Politics of Education*, 32(2), 217–234.

Lister, R. (1990). Women, economic dependency and citizenship. *Journal of Social Policy*, 19(04), 445–467.

Lister, R. (2004). *Poverty*. Cambridge: Polity Press.

Lister, R., and Bennett, F. (2010). The new 'champion of progressive ideals'? *Renewal: A Journal of Labour Politics*, 18(1/2), 84.

Livesey, R. (2004). Reading for character: women social reformers and narratives of the urban poor in late Victorian and Edwardian London. *Journal of Victorian Culture*, 9(1), 43–67.

Locke, J. (1697) [1997]. An essay on the Poor Law. In M. Goldie (ed.) *Locke: Political Essays*. Cambridge: Cambridge University Press.

Ludwig, J., Duncan, G. J., Gennetian, L. A., Katz, L. F., Kessler, R. C., Kling, J. R., and Sanbonmatsu, L. (2012). Neighborhood effects on the long-term well-being of low-income adults. *Science*, 337(6101), 1505–1510.

Lupton, R. (2003). *Poverty Street: The Dynamics of Neighbourhood Decline and Renewal*. Bristol: Policy Press.

MacLeavy, J. (2011). A 'new politics' of austerity, workfare and gender? The UK coalition government's welfare reform proposals. *Cambridge Journal of Regions, Economy and Society*, 4(3), 355–367.

Malanima, P. (2005). Urbanisation and the Italian economy during the last millennium. *European Review of Economic History*, 9(1), 97–122.

Malthus, T. R. (1798) [1805]. *An Essay on the Principle of Population*. London: J. Johnson.

Manji, K. (2016). Social security reform and the surveillance state: exploring the operation of 'hidden conditionality' in the reform of disability benefits since 2010. *Social Policy and Society*. doi:10.1017/S147474641600052X.

Manley, D., Van Ham, M., and Doherty, J. (2012). Social mixing as a cure for negative neighbourhood effects: evidence-based policy or urban myth. In G. Bridge, T. Butler, and L. Lees (eds) *Mixed Communities: Gentrification by Stealth?* Bristol: Policy Press.

Manzi, T. (2015). The big society and the conjunction of crises: justifying welfare reform and undermining social housing. *Housing, Theory and Society*, 32(1), 9–24.

Marcuse, P. (1996). Space and race in the post-fordist city: the outcast ghetto and advanced homelessness in the United States today. In E. Mingione (ed.) *Urban Poverty and the Underclass: A Reader*. Oxford: Blackwell.

Marcuse, P. (1997). The ghetto of exclusion and the fortified enclave: new patterns in the United States. *American Behavioral Scientist*, 41(3), 311–326.

Marcuse, P. (2005). Enclaves yes, ghettos no: segregation and the state. In D. P. Varady (ed.) *Desegregating the City: Ghettos, Enclaves, and Inequality*. New York: State University of New York Press.

Marshall, T. H. (1950). *Citizenship and Social Class, and Other Essays*. Cambridge: Cambridge University Press.

Martz, L. (1983). *Poverty and Welfare in Habsburg Spain*. Cambridge: Cambridge University Press.

Marx, K. (1887). *Capital: A Critique of Political Economy, Vol. 1*. Harmondsworth: Penguin.

Massey, D. S. (2007). *Categorically Unequal: The American Stratification System*. New York: Russell Sage Foundation.

Massey, D. S., and Denton, N. A. (1989). Hypersegregation in US metropolitan areas: black and Hispanic segregation along five dimensions. *Demography*, 26(3), 373–391.

Massey, D. S., and Tannen, J. (2015). A research note on trends in black hyper-segregation. *Demography*, 52(3), 1025–1034.

Matsaganis, M., Ferrera, M., Capucha, L., and Moreno, L. (2003). Mending Nets in the South: Anti-poverty Policies in Greece, Italy, Portugal and Spain. *Social Policy and Administration*, 37(6), 639–655.

Mau, S. (2003). *The Moral Economy of Welfare States: Britain and Germany Compared*. London and New York: Routledge.

Mauss, M. (1954). *Forms and Functions of Exchange in Archaic Society*. Glencoe: the Free Press.

Mazumdar, P. M. (1980). The eugenists and the residuum: the problem of the urban poor. *Bulletin of the History of Medicine*, 54(2), 204–215.

McCord, N. (1976). The Poor Law and philanthropy. In D. Fraser (ed.) *The New Poor Law in the Nineteenth Century*. London and Basingstoke: Macmillan.

McCormack, K. (2004). Resisting the welfare mother: the power of welfare discourse and tactics of resistance. *Critical Sociology*, 30(2), 355–383.

McIntosh, M. (2012). *Poor Relief in England, 1350–1600*. Cambridge: Cambridge University Press.

McLaughlin, D. K., Stokes, C. S., Smith, P. J., and Nonoyama, A. (2007). Differential mortality across the United States: the influence of place-based inequality. In L. M. Lobao, G. Hooks, and A. R. Tickamyer (eds) *The Sociology of Spatial Inequality*. Albany: State University of New York Press.

McMullan, J. L. (1987). Crime, law and order in early modern England. *British Journal of Criminology*, 27(3), 252–274.

Merton, R. K. (1948). The self-fulfilling prophecy. *Antioch Review*, 8(2), 193–210.

Merton, R. K. (1972). Insiders and outsiders: a chapter in the sociology of knowledge. *American Journal of Sociology*, 78(1), 9–47.

Milanovic, B. (1995). *Poverty, Inequality, and Social Policy in Transition Economies*. Washington, DC: World Bank.

Mill, J. S. (1865). *Auguste Comte and Positivism*. Ann Arbor: University of Michigan Press.

Miller Jr, R. A. (1974). Are familists amoral? A test of Banfield's amoral familism hypothesis in a south Italian village. *American Ethnologist*, 1(3), 515–535.

Mingione, E. (1996). Conclusions. In E. Mingione (ed.) *Urban Poverty and the Underclass: A Reader*. Cambridge, MA: Blackwell.

Mishra, R. (1984). *The Welfare State in Crisis: Social Thought and Social Change*. Brighton: Wheatsheaf.

Moffatt, S., and Noble, E. (2015). Work or welfare after cancer? Explorations of identity and stigma. *Sociology of Health and Illness*, 37(8), 1191–1205.

Mooney, G. (2011). *Stigmatising poverty? The 'Broken Society' and Reflections on Anti-Welfarism in the UK Today*. Oxford: Oxfam.

Morawska, E. (2009). *A Sociology of Immigration: (Re)Making Multifaceted America*. Basingstoke: Palgrave Macmillan.

Morichini, C. L. (1870). *Degli istituti di carità per la sussistenza e l'educazione dei poveri e dei prigionieri in Roma*. Roma: Stabilimento Tipografico Camerale.

Morini, C. (1995). Xenodochium nelle Glosse Anglosassoni ai 'Bella Parisiacae Urbis' di Abbone di St. Germain-des-Prés. *Aevum*, 69(2), 347–355.

Morley, N. (2006). The poor in the city of Rome. In M. Atkins and R. Osborne (eds) *Poverty in the Roman World*. Cambridge and New York: Cambridge University Press.

Morlicchio, E., and Pugliese, E. (2006). Naples: unemployment and spatial exclusion. In S. Musterd, A. Murie, and C. Kesteloot (eds) *Neighbourhoods of Poverty: Urban Social Exclusion and Integration in Europe*. Basingstoke: Palgrave Macmillan.

Morlicchio, E., Pugliese, E., and Spinelli, E. (2002). Diminishing welfare: the Italian case. In G. S. Goldberg and M. G. Rosenthal (eds), *Diminishing Welfare: A Cross-National Study of Social Provision*. Westport, CT and London: Greenwood.

Morris, L. (2002). *Dangerous Classes: The Underclass and Social Citizenship*. Abingdon: Routledge.

Muraskin, W., (1974). The moral basis of a backward sociologist: Edward Banfield, the Italians, and the Italian-Americans. *American Journal of Sociology*, 79(6), 1484–1496.

Moscovici, S. (1988). Notes towards a description of social representations. *European Journal of Social Psychology*, 18(3), 211–250.

Moskoff, W. (1992). *Unemployment in the Soviet Union*. Washington, DC: National Council for Soviet and East European Research.

Mowat, C. L. (1961). *The Charity Organisation Society, 1869–1913: Its Ideas and Work*. Edinburgh: Constable.

Muratori, L. A. (1723). *Della carità cristiana, in quanto essa è amore del prossimo*. Modena: Bartolomeo Soliani.

Murray, C. A. (1984). *Losing Ground: American Social Policy, 1950–1980*. New York: Basic Books.

Musterd, S. (2005). Social and ethnic segregation in Europe: levels, causes, and effects. *Journal of Urban Affairs*, 27(3), 331–348.

Naldini, M. (2004). *The Family in the Mediterranean Welfare States*. Abingdon: Routledge.

Newman, C. (2014). To Punish or Protect: The New Poor Law and the English Workhouse. *International Journal of Historical Archaeology*, 18(1), 122–145.

Niceforo, A. (1908). *Antropologia delle classi povere*. Milano: Vallardi.

Nicoloso, P. (1995). L'albergo dei poveri di Palermo. In A.Guerra, E. Molteni, and P. Nicoloso (eds) *Il trionfo della miseria. Gli alberghi dei poveri di Genova, Palermo e Napoli*. Milano: Electa.

Nye, R. A. (1985). The bio-medical origins of urban sociology. *Journal of Contemporary History*, 20(4), 659–675.

O'Connor, J. (1973). *The Fiscal Crisis of the Welfare State*. New York: St Martin's.

O'Connor, A. (2002). *Poverty Knowledge: Social Science, Social Policy and the Poor in Twentieth-Century U.S. History*. Princeton: Princeton University Press.

Orford, S., Dorling, D., Mitchell, R., Shaw, M., and Smith, G. D. (2002). Life and death of the people of London: a historical GIS of Charles Booth's inquiry. *Health and Place*, 8(1), 25–35.

Ostendorf, W., Musterd, S., and De Vos, S. (2001). Social mix and the neighbourhood effect. policy ambitions and empirical evidence. *Housing Studies*, 16(3), 371–380.

Östh, J., Malmberg, B., and Andersson, E. K. (2015). Analysing segregation using individualised neighbourhoods. In C. D. Lloyd, I. G. Shuttleworth, and D. W. Wong (eds) *Social–Spatial Segregation: Concepts, Processes and Outcomes*. Bristol: Policy Press.

Paci, M., and Pugliese, E. (eds) (2011). *Welfare e promozione delle capacità*. Bologna: Mulino.

Page, R. M. (1996). *Altruism and the British Welfare State*. Aldershot: Avebury.

Palen, J. J., and London, B. (eds) (1984). *Gentrification, Displacement, and Neighborhood Revitalization*. Albany: State University of New York Press.

Pardo, I. (1996). *Managing Existence in Naples: Morality, Action and Structure*. Cambridge: Cambridge University Press.

Patrick, R. (2014). Welfare reform and the valorisation of work: is work really the best form of welfare? In M. Harrison and T. Sanders (eds) *Social Policies and Social Control: New Perspectives on the 'Not-So-Big Society'*. Bristol: Policy Press.

Patrick, R., and Brown, K. (2012). Re-moralising or de-moralising? *People, Place and Policy Online*, 6(1), 1–4.

Paugam, S., and Selz, M. (2005). La perception de la pauvreté en Europe depuis le milieu des années 1970. Analyse des variations structurelles et conjoncturelles. *Économie et statistique*, 383(1), 283–305.

Paugam, S. (2009). What forms does poverty take in European societies at the beginning of the twenty-first century? In K. De Boyser, C. Dewilde, D. Dierckx, and J. Friedrichs (eds) *Between the Social and the Spatial: Exploring the Multiple Dimensions of Poverty and Social Exclusion*. Farnham: Ashgate.

Paul, D. (1984). Eugenics and the left. *Journal of the History of Ideas*, 45(4), 567–590.

Paz-Fuchs, A. (2008). Behind the contract for welfare reform: antecedent themes in welfare to work programs. *Berkeley Journal of Employment and Labor Law*, 29(2), 405–454.

Peach, C. (1996). Does Britain have ghettos? *Transactions of the Institute of British Geographers*, 21(1), 216–235.

Peach, C. (2005). The ghetto and the ethnic enclave. In D. P. Varady (ed.) *Desegregating the City: Ghettos, Enclaves, and Inequality*. Albany: State University of New York Press.

Peach, C. (2009). Slippery segregation: discovering or manufacturing ghettos? *Journal of Ethnic and Migration Studies*, 35(9), 1381–1395.

Pellissery, S., Lødemel, I., and Gubrium, E. K. (2014). Shame and shaming in policy processes. In E. K. Gubrium, S. Pellissery, and I. Lødemel (eds) *The Shame of It: Global Perspectives on Anti-Poverty Policies*. Bristol: Policy Press.

Petersen, M. B., Slothuus, R., Stubager, R., and Togeby, L. (2010). Deservingness versus values in public opinion on welfare: the automaticity of the deservingness heuristic. *European Journal of Political Research*, 50(1), 24–52.

Petitti di Roreto, C. I. (1837). *Saggio sul buon governo della mendicità, degli istituti di beneficenza e delle carceri*. Torino: Bocca.

Picton, C. (1975). Beyond the stereotype: another view of supplementary benefits officers. *British Journal of Social Work*, 5(4), 441–457.

Pierson, P. (1994). *Dismantling the Welfare State? Reagan, Thatcher and the Politics of Retrenchment*. Cambridge: Cambridge University Press.

Pierson, P. (1996). The new politics of the welfare state. *World Politics*, 48, 143–179.

Piven, F. F., and Cloward, R. (1971). *Regulating the Poor: The Functions of Public Welfare*. New York: Vintage.

Polanyi, K. (1944) [1957]. *The Great Transformation: The Political and Economic Origins of Our Times*. Boston: Beacon.

Pound, J. F. (1971) [2013]. *Poverty and Vagrancy in Tudor England*. London and New York: Routledge.

Powell, M. A. (2008). *Modernising the Welfare State: The Blair Legacy*. Bristol: Policy Press.

Poynter, J. R. (1969). *Society and Pauperism: English Ideas on Poor Relief, 1795–1834*. Melbourne: Melbourne University Press.

Prochaska, F. (1988). *The Voluntary Impulse: Philanthropy in Modern Britain*. London: Faber.

Pullan, B. (1976). Catholics and the poor in early modern Europe. *Transactions of the Royal Historical Society*, 26, 15–34.

Pullan, B. (1988). Support and redeem: charity and poor relief in Italian cities from the fourteenth to the seventeenth century. *Continuity and Change*, 3(2), 177–208.

Pullan, B. (1995). Introduction. In A. Guerra, E. Molteni, and P. Nicoloso (eds) *Il trionfo della miseria. Gli alberghi dei poveri di Genova, Palermo e Napoli*. Milano: Electa.

Pullan, B. (2005). Catholics, Protestants, and the poor in early modern Europe. *Journal of Interdisciplinary History*, 35(3), 441–456.

Putnam, B. H. (1908). *The Enforcement of the Statutes of Labourers during the First Decade after the Black Death, 1349–1359*. New York: Columbia University Press.

Quadagno, J. (1994). *The Color of Welfare: How Racism Undermined the War on Poverty*. Oxford: Oxford University Press.

Quine, M. S. (2002). *Italy's Social Revolution: Charity and Welfare from Liberalism to Fascism*. Basingstoke: Palgrave Macmillan.

Ranci, C. (1994). The third sector in welfare policies in Italy: The contradictions of a protected market. *Voluntas: International Journal of Voluntary and Nonprofit Organizations*, 5(3), 247–271.

Ranci, C., and Migliavacca, M. (2015). Main policy changes in the Italian welfare state over the past two decades. In U. Ascoli and E. Pavolini (eds) *The Italian Welfare State in a European Perspective: A Comparative Analysis*. Bristol: Policy Press.

Rawlings, P. (2002). *Policing: A Short History*. Cullompton: Willan.

Rhee, H. (2012). *Loving the Poor, Saving the Rich: Wealth, Poverty, and Early Christian Formation*. Grand Rapids, MI: Baker.

Rhodes, M. (ed.) (1997). *Southern European Welfare States: Between Crisis and Reform*. London: Frank Cass.

Rimlinger, G. V. (1961). Social Security, Incentives, and Controls in the U.S. and U.S. S.R. *Comparative Studies in Society and History*, 4(1), 104–124.

Roof, M. (1957). *Voluntary Societies and Social Policy*. London: Routledge & Kegan Paul.

Roof, M. (1972). *A Hundred Years of Family Welfare: A Study of the Family Welfare Association (Formerly Charity Organisation Society) 1869–1969*. London: Michael Joseph.

Rose, G. (1805). *Observations on the Poor laws, and on the management of the poor, in Great Britain arising from a consideration of the returns now before Parliament*. London: J. Hatchard.

Rose, M., and Baumgartner, F. R. (2013). Framing the poor: media coverage and US poverty policy, 1960–2008. *Policy Studies Journal*, 4(1), 22–53.

Rose, M. E. (1972). *The Relief of Poverty, 1834–1914*. London and Basingstoke: Macmillan.

Rowntree, B. S. (1901). *Poverty: A Study of Town Life*. London: Macmillan.

Russo Krauss, D. (2014). Some considerations about spatial concentration and segregation of immigrants in Naples. *Documenti Geografici*, 2, 113–124.

Sanders, T. (2014). Concluding thoughts: the consequence of a 'not-so-big society'. In M. Harrison and T. Sanders (eds) *Social Policies and Social Control: New Perspectives on the 'Not-So-Big Society'*. Bristol: Policy Press.

Saraceno, C. (1990). Women, family, and the law, 1750–1942. *Journal of Family History*, 15(4), 427–442.

Saraceno, C. (1991). Dalla istituzionalizzazione alla de-istituzionalizzazione dei corsi di vita femminili e maschili? *Stato e mercato*, 33(3), 431–449.

Saraceno, C. (1994). The ambivalent familism of the Italian welfare state. *Social Politics: International Studies in Gender, State and Society*, 1(1), 60–82.

Saraceno, C. (2002). *Social Assistance Dynamics in Europe: National and Local Poverty Regimes*. Bristol: Policy Press.

Saraceno, C. (2010). Social inequalities in facing old-age dependency: a bi-generational perspective. *Journal of European Social Policy*, 20(1), 32–44.

Saraceno, C., and Keck, W. (2010). Can we identify intergenerational policy regimes in Europe? *European Societies*, 12(5), 675–696.

Saraceno, C., and Negri, N. (1994). The changing Italian welfare state. *Journal of European Social Policy*, 4(1), 19–34.

Saunders, P. (2013). *Re-moralising the Welfare State*. St Leonards, NSW: Centre for Independent Studies.

Scaglia, E. (1863). *Manuale per le amministrazioni di beneficenza ossia la legge 3 agosto 1862 ed il regolamento 27 successivo novembre sulle Opere pie*. Torino: Tipografia Nazionale di G. Biancardi.

Schmidt, V. A. (2001). The politics of economic adjustment in France and Britain: when does discourse matter? *Journal of European Public Policy*, 8(2), 247–264.

Schmidtz, D., and Goodin, R. E. (1998). *Social Welfare and Individual Responsibility*. Cambridge: Cambridge University Press

Schneider, A. L., and Ingram, H. (eds) (2005). *Deserving and Entitled: Social Constructions and Public Policy*. Albany: State University of New York Press.

Scull, A. (1980). 'Moral Architecture. The Victorian Lunatic Asylum'. In A. D. King (ed.) *Buildings and Society. Essays in the Social Development of the Built Environment*, London and Boston: Routledge and Kegan Paul.

Searle, G. R. (1998). *Morality and the Market in Victorian Britain*. Oxford: Clarendon.

Semyonov, M., and Herring, C. (2007). Segregated jobs or ethnic niches? The impact of racialized employment on earnings inequality. *Research in Social Stratification and Mobility*, 25(4), 245–257.

Sen, A. (1992). *Inequality Re-Examined*. Cambridge, MA: Harvard University Press.

Seyd, P. (1976). The Child Poverty Action Group. *Political Quarterly*, 47(2), 189–202.

Shildrick, T., MacDonald, R., and Webster, C. (2012). *Poverty and Insecurity: Life In 'Low-Pay, No-Pay' Britain*. Bristol: Policy Press.

Silvano, G. (2007). Pathways to the contemporary Italian welfare state. In G. Hagemann (ed.) *Reciprocity and Redistribution: Work and Welfare Reconsidered*. Pisa: Edizioni Plus.

Silverman, S. F. (1968). Agricultural organization, social structure, and values in Italy: amoral familism reconsidered. *American Anthropologist*, 70(1), 1–20.

Simmel, G., and Jacobson, C. (1965). The poor. *Social Problems*, 13(2), 118–140.

Smith, N. (1996). *The New Urban Frontier: Gentrification and the Revanchist City*. New York and London: Routledge.

Smith, S. R. (1997). Disarming the ideological conflict between the centre-left and the new right: the implementation of UK social security policy. *Journal of Political Ideologies*, 2(1), 79–97.

Smithson, J. (2008). Focus groups. In P. Alasuutari, L. Bickman, and J. Brannen (eds). *The SAGE Handbook of Social Research Methods*. London: Sage.

Speizman, M. D. (1966). Speenhamland: an experiment in guaranteed income. *Social Service Review*, 40(1), 44–55.

Spicker, P. (2007). *The Idea of Poverty*. Bristol: Policy Press.

Spicker, P. (2013a). Liberal welfare states. In B. Greve (ed.) *The Routledge Handbook of the Welfare State*. London and New York: Routledge.

Spicker, P. (2013b). *Reclaiming Individualism*. Bristol: Policy Press.

Steensland, B. (2010). Moral classification and social policy. In S. Hitlin and S. Vaisey (eds) *Handbook of the Sociology of Morality*. New York: Springer.

Szelenyi, I. (1983). *Urban Inequalities under State Socialism*. Oxford: Oxford University Press.

Taylor, A. J. (1972). *Laissez-Faire and State Intervention in Nineteenth-Century Britain*. London: Macmillan.

Terranova, T. (2004). Communication beyond meaning: on the cultural politics of information. *Social Text*, 22(3), 51–73.

Thomas, W. I., and Thomas, D. S. (1928) [1970]. *The Child in America: Behavior Problems and Programs.* New York: Knopf.

Thompson, E. P. (1971). The moral economy of the English crowd in the eighteenth century. *Past and Present*, 50(1971), 76–136.

Titmuss, R. M. (1950). *Problems of Social Policy.* London: HMSO.

Titmuss, R. M. (1974). *Social Policy.* London: Allen & Unwin.

Townsend, P. (1962). The Meaning of Poverty. *British Journal of Sociology*, 13(3), 210–227.

Tronrud, T. J. (1985). The response to poverty in three English towns, 1560–1640: a comparative approach. *Histoire sociale/Social History*, 18(35), 9–27.

Valentino, N. A., Hutchings, V. L., and White, I. K. (2002). Cues that matter: how political ads prime racial attitudes during campaigns. *American Political Science Review*, 96(1), 75–90.

Van der Laan Bouma-Doff, W. (2007). Involuntary isolation: Ethnic preferences and residential segregation. *Journal of Urban Affairs*, 29(3), 289–309.

Van Ham, M., and Manley, D. (2015). Segregation, choice based letting and social housing: how housing policy can affect the segregation process. In C. D. Lloyd, I. G. Shuttleworth, and D. W. Wong (eds) *Social–Spatial Segregation: Concepts, Processes and Outcomes.* Bristol: Policy Press.

Van Kempen, R. (2005). Segregation and housing conditions of immigrants in Western European cities. In Y. Kazepov (ed.) *Cities of Europe: Changing Contexts, Local Arrangements, and the Challenge to Urban Cohesion.* Malden, MA and Oxford: Blackwell.

Van Kempen, R., and Şule Özüekren, A. (1998). Ethnic segregation in cities: new forms and explanations in a dynamic world. *Urban Studies*, 35(10), 1631–1656.

Van Oorschot, W., Opielka, M., and Pfau-Effinger, B. (eds) (2008). *Culture and Welfare State: Values and Social Policy in Comparative Perspective.* Cheltenham: Edward Elgar.

Van Til, K. A. (2010). Poverty and morality in Christianity. In W. A. Galston and P. H. Hoffenberg (eds) *Poverty and Morality: Religious and Secular Perspectives.* Cambridge: Cambridge University Press.

Veit-Wilson, J. H. (1992). Muddle or mendacity? The Beveridge Committee and the poverty line. *Journal of Social Policy*, 21(03), 269–301.

Vincent, A. W. (1984). The Poor Law reports of 1909 and the social theory of the Charity Organization Society . *Victorian Studies*, 27(3), 343–363.

Wacquant, L. (2009). *Punishing the Poor: The Neoliberal Government of Social Insecurity.* Durham, NC and London: Duke University Press.

Wacquant, L. J. D. (1993). Urban outcasts: stigma and division in the black American ghetto and the French urban periphery. *International Journal of Urban and Regional Research*, 17(3), 366–383.

Wacquant, L. J. D. (1996). The rise of advanced marginality: notes on its nature and implications. *Acta sociologica*, 39(2), 121–139.

Wacquant, L. J. D. (1998). Urban marginality in the coming millennium. *Urban Studies*, 36(10), 1639–1647.

Wacquant, L. J. D. (2007). French working-class banlieues and black American ghetto: from conflation to comparison. *Qui parle*, 16(2), 5–38.

Wacquant, L. J. D., and Wilson, W. J. (1993). The cost of racial and class exclusion in the inner city. In W. J. Wilson (ed.) *The Ghetto Underclass: Social Science Perspectives.* London: Sage.

Wallace, A. (2014). New Labour, the coalition government and disciplined communities. In M. Harrison and T. Sanders, *Social Policies and Social Control: New Perspectives on the 'Not-So-Big Society'*. Bristol: Policy Press.

Wardhaugh, J. (2000). *Sub City: Young People, Homelessness and Crime*. Aldershot: Ashgate.

Webb, S. (1910). Eugenics and the Poor Law. The Minority Report. *Eugenics Review*, 2(3), 233–241.

Webb, S. (1928). *The English Poor Law: Will It Endure?* London: Oxford University Press.

Webb, S., and Webb, B. (1911). *The Prevention of Destitution*. London: Longman, Green & Co.

Weber, L., and Bowling, B. (2008). Valiant beggars and global vagabonds: select, eject, immobilize. *Theoretical Criminology*, 12(3), 355–375.

Weber, M. (1930) [2005]. *The Protestant Ethic and the Spirit of Capitalism*. London and New York: Routledge.

Weinbren, D., and James, B. (2005). Getting a grip: the roles of friendly societies in Australia and Britain reappraised. *Labour History*, 88, 87–103.

Weiner, B., Osborne, D., and Rudolph, U. (2011). An attributional analysis of reactions to poverty: the political ideology of the giver and the perceived morality of the receiver. *Personality and Social Psychology Review*, 15(2), 199–213.

Whelan, R. (2001). *Helping the Poor: Friendly Visiting, Dole Charities and Dole Queues*. London: Civitas.

Whittington, C. (1977). Social workers' orientations: an action perspective. *British Journal of Social Work*, 7(1), 73–95.

Wiener, M. J. (1990). *Reconstructing the Criminal: Culture, Law, and Policy in England, 1830–1914*. Cambridge: Cambridge University Press.

Wiles, P. J. D., and Markowski, S. (1971). Income Distribution under Communism and Capitalism: Some Facts about Poland, the UK, the USA and the USSR. *Soviet Studies*, 22(4), 487–511.

Wilkes, R., and Iceland, J. (2004). Hypersegregation in the twenty-first century. *Demography*, 41(1), 23–36.

Williams, A., Goodwin, M., and Cloke, P. (2014). Neoliberalism, Big Society, and progressive localism. *Environment and Planning*, 46(12), 2798–2815.

Williams, K. (1981). *From Pauperism to Poverty*. London: Routledge & Kegan Paul.

Wilson, W. J. (1978). *The Declining Significance of Race: Blacks and Changing American Institutions*. Chicago and London: University of Chicago Press.

Wilson, W. J. (1987). *The Truly Disadvantaged: The Inner City, the Underclass, and Public Policy*. Chicago and London: University of Chicago Press.

Wilson, W. J. (1988). The ghetto underclass and the social transformation of the inner city. *The Black Scholar*, 19(3), 10–17.

Wirth, L. (1927). The ghetto. *American Journal of Sociology*, 33(1), 57–71.

Wirth, L. (1928). *The Ghetto*. London and Chicago: University of Chicago Press.

Wissink, B., Schwanen, T., and Van Kempen, R. (2016). Beyond residential segregation: Introduction. *Cities*, 59, 126–130.

Woodbridge, L. (2001). *Vagrancy, Homelessness, and English Renaissance Literature*. Urbana and Chicago: University of Illinois Press.

Woods, R. A. (1914). The neighborhood in social reconstruction. *American Journal of Sociology*, 19(5), 577–591.

Woodward, S. L. (1995). *Socialist Unemployment: The Political Economy of Yugoslavia, 1945–1990*. Princeton: Princeton University Press.

Woolf, S. (1991). The poor and how to relieve them: The Restoration debate on poverty in Italy and Europe. In A. Davis and P. Ginsborg (eds) *Society and Politics in the Age of the Risorgimento: Essays in Honour of Denis Mack Smith*. Cambridge: Cambridge University Press.

Zubkova, Y. (2010). Marginal population groups and state policy, 1940s–1960s. *Social Sciences*, 41(2), 13–34.

Index